I0222728

Collagen

Effective Recipes to Improve Strengthen Joints

(Most Effective Step by Step Guide for Beginners)

Robert Tan

Published By **Andrew Zen**

Robert Tan

All Rights Reserved

Collagen: Effective Recipes to Improve Strengthen Joints (Most Effective Step by Step Guide for Beginners)

ISBN   978-1-77485-778-6

No part of this guidebook shall be reproduced in any form without permission in writing from the publisher except in the case of brief quotations embodied in critical articles or reviews.

Legal & Disclaimer

The information contained in this ebook is not designed to replace or take the place of any form of medicine or professional medical advice. The information in this ebook has been provided for educational & entertainment purposes only.

The information contained in this book has been compiled from sources deemed reliable, and it is accurate to the best of the Author's knowledge; however, the Author cannot guarantee its accuracy and validity and cannot be held liable for any errors or omissions. Changes are periodically made to this book. You must consult your doctor or get professional medical advice before using any of the suggested remedies, techniques, or information in this book.

Upon using the information contained in this book, you agree to hold harmless the Author from and against any damages, costs, and expenses, including any legal fees potentially resulting from the application of any of the information provided by this guide. This disclaimer applies to any damages or injury caused by the use and application, whether directly or indirectly, of any advice or information presented, whether for breach of contract, tort, negligence, personal injury, criminal intent, or under any other cause of action.

You agree to accept all risks of using the information presented inside this book. You need to consult a professional medical practitioner in order to ensure you are both able and healthy enough to participate in this program.

Table Of Contents

Introduction

Are you wondering why your skin remains firm and youthful and loosens as we the passage of
It's caused by collagen or a lack of it.
Collagen is fibrous protein that provides our skin with its elasticity and firmness. It also replaces dead skin cells within our bodies. Collagen has a major part to play in the way we appear and feel since it is a significant part of 30 percent of our body's protein. The term Collagen is derived from an ancient Greek word"kolla" (kolla) that translates as "glue". A fitting word for something that helps to hold our body in place. And it holds us together. does, because it is that strong, one gram of Type 1 collagen fibrils' can be more powerful than the same weight of steel.
Type I collagen is among the highest-quality protein throughout the human body. It's found in muscles joints and blood vessels, tendons as well as skin, bones and even in the digestive tract. However, there's a catch: after just 25

years, our body's collagen production begins to slow at the rate of 1.5 percent annually. Thus, around the age of 25 we reach our peak. When this production slows the body's fibers are brittle and begin to disintegrate, resulting in a variety of negative effects of aging.

It's not only about getting younger-looking skin. The collagen tale is about having strong bones and the ability to do more through an improved body. This book will take a look at the research that supports the benefits of consumption and use of collagen as a way to improve the appearance and strength of hair, skin, teeth, nails and bones. We will also look at different types of collagen and the best ways to make lasting changes to enhance health and well-being.

Chapter 1: Collagen

"Zest" is the key ingredient to all beauty. There isn't a beauty that is appealing without zest."

- Christian Dior

The most nutritious food source is nature, regardless of what the marketing departments try to inform us. One of the most important areas in nutrition and nutrition science is proteins, specifically, how can we consume and utilize protein effectively to enhance our overall health.

This book is about a specific type of protein: collagen. Collagen is an organic, digestible and bioactive protein that is produced by bovine, porcine and chicken as well as marine cells. It is an extremely effective type of protein, and is utilized to increase the strength of bones as well as appearance and health of teeth, hair skin, and nails.

At the end of this book, you'll know why collagen is vital to our diets, particularly for those who are over 25. The research that supports collagen supplements' claims for health benefits as well as the options that you can choose from when making use of collagen.

There are many technical terms that are useful in this book The definitions are as the following:

* Peptides - - Peptides contain chains of amino acid which constitute the basic building blocks of skin-related proteins. They can penetrate the upper layers of the skin, and send signals to cells that tell them how to perform.

* Muscles are made up of protein and contain lots of protein. After digestion, it breaks to amino acids. These amino acids may then be used to make new proteins. Proteins play a significant role in food items like eggs, milk and meat, as well as beans, fish, pulses and nuts.

* Amino Acid * Amino Acid Amino acids bind together to form long chains. The lengthy chains made of amino acids can be known as proteins.

* Hydrolysis - Hydrolysis refers to an reaction in chemistry or that occurs when

a chemical compound is reacted with water. This is the kind of reaction used to break polymers into smaller pieces.

* Hydrolysed Protein - a protein that is hydrolyzed and broken into components amino acids.

The technical aspect is that collagen peptides consist of three polypeptide chains that are wrapped around each other to create triple-helical macromolecules, unique amino acid sequence. This sequence is crucial in assembling the fibrils that create fibres and ensure structure and strength for your conjunctive tissues.

What this means for you can be that collagen-peptides serve as an important protein that helps the body in order to maintain hair, teeth, joint and overall health of the skin.

What are the various forms of collagen?

Perhaps you've seen collagen supplements, or perhaps gelatin is a type of gelatin that can aid in improving your skin's health as well as condition and moisturize your hair. make your nails have a more natural shine. There are several kinds of collagen, such as Type 1 and Type 2 and Type 3. They contain various proteins that all are involved in the workings of the body. They can be explained in the following manner:

Type I collagen

Like other collagens Type 1 collagen is the triple helix, which comprises three strands. Each strand measures around 300 nanometers long , and it has 1050 amino acids. Hydrogen is present between amino acids as well as the strands binding them and enhancing the strength of the fiber massively.

The type I collagen can be very sturdy and is the most important component of tendon. It also aids in strengthening bones.

Type II collagen

This kind of collagen is the primary component of cartilage. Cartilage is the tough connective tissue found in the nose, ears and various joints of the body. They strengthen cartilage and provide durability.

Type II fibrils tend to be smaller than their counterparts of type I. The type II collagen made through the matrix non-cellular that forms part of cartilage.

Type III collagen

While it's not as sturdy as Type I collagen, over 90% of your body's collagen is composed from collagen of Type I or III collagen. These are composed of proteins like proline, hydroxyprolineand alanine and Glycine. Collagen Type III can be usually found in the arterial walls in intestines, the gastrointestinal tract and, of course, on the skin. It also makes triple helices, which are full of strength too. This type of collagen is renowned because of its capacity to seal damaged skin. This is because the body makes this kind of collagen much faster than other kind of collagen. This is why, once the wound is allowed to heal it is when the body replaces the type III collagen using type I which is then used to create scar tissue.

The production of collagen by the body is at its peak around the 20s, but shortly afterward, it begins to decrease. In the process, our skin gets thinner, less firm, and begins to form deep wrinkles and sagging.

For the modern-day consumer, it's not a secret the fact that collagen in good health help to give you young skin. The best way to keep healthy collagen levels is to guard the collagen that is already in our bodies. This can be achieved by avoiding sun exposure as well as taking collagen supplements in all of the above forms. The product is advertised as anti-aging collagen formulations are receiving lots of attention from the beauty business. Females in Japan have been drinking collagen liquid for a long time to obtain young, smooth, and firm skin. However, European and Americans are just beginning to be conscious of the advantages of collagen.

Collagen supplements and other beauty products are available in the form of tablets, liquids, powders capsules, soft chewables , etc. The supplements are usually composed of animal extracts, that is derived from cow, chicken or pig. The collagen from fish extract is believed to be the best as it appears that the body is able to absorb it more efficiently due to its small molecular weight.

Supplements that have type I or III can:

* Improve skin elasticity

* Reducing the appearance of wrinkles as well as fine lines.

Reduce hair loss and increase volume

* Give support to the bone matrix

* Repair damaged nail bed

* Increase the production of glycine and assist in the development of stronger strong muscles

* Help burn fat during sleep

Type II collagen supplements may:

* Increase the content of cartilage's protein with

* Increase the protein content of cartilage articular

* Reduce popping knees

* Might help strengthen joints as well as jaw

The length of time it takes to see the advantages of collagen supplements could differ. Most people see the results begin to show after just a few weeks after the intake however for some it could take months.

Keep in mind that all collagen supplements aren't all created to be the same. If the collagen supplement you are taking isn't properly absorbed into your body by the body's system, it will not give you any outcomes.

Is collagen protein? What distinguishes it from other proteins?

Collagen is a naturally occurring skin-friendly protein used by thousands of people to fight the signs of aging. Certain cells in our bodies like fibroblasts create collagen proteins in the form procollagen. When procollagen is released by cells it produces active collagen that binds with each other to form fibrils.

Collagen is an extremely complex molecule, that the human body can't absorb in its original state. It's simply too big to be absorbed by the skin by lotions and other products. And due to this same factor, the stomach isn't able to disintegrate it quickly. This is why it's always changing through cosmetics as well as health supplements companies to help make it more absorbable and this leads to many different types of cosmetics and supplements you've been able to find in the marketplace.

Now that we have this in mind we'll move to chapter 2, where we will discuss the many advantages of Collagen together with the collagen pills and creams.

Chapter 2: The Benefits Of Collagen

"The quest for beauty and truth is a realm of action
where we are allowed to
We will always be children."
Albert Einstein

Collagen is crucial for well-being of joints, bones tissues, joints, and skin. As well as helping to keep the skin flawless and firm as well as helping to smooth the skin tone. It's also important to reduce the various signs of aging. At the age of 25 the body's collagen production diminishes and leads to the process of aging to accelerate. The body's regular supply of collagen could slow down the process.

Although many people are aware of the well-known advantages, there's plenty more that collagen has to offer. With its many advantages, collagen has recently been introduced to grocery stores for health foods and on the shelves of the kitchen of those who are health conscious. Benefits of collagen vary from easing joints to lessen wrinkles, improving digestion and many more. Here's how collagen helps.

#1 - Repairs Joints , Connective Tissue

Joint injuries take an extended amount of time to recover. In addition to taking plenty of rest and allowing it to heal, one can aid the body to repair the injuries from the inside. This will aid in repairing the integrity of connective tissues. Collagen decreases inflammation, and may even treat degenerative diseases like osteoarthritis.

#2 - Enhances Skin Health

Collagen is composed mainly of amino acids such as proline, glycine and proline hydroxyproline. These amino acids help reduce signs of ageing and encourage youthful looking skin. Collagen is the essential ingredient for the regeneration that takes place on the face. It provides the smoothness, elasticity, cohesion and suppleness. It also improves the skin's moisture levels.

Incorporating collagen in your diet will reduce the appearance of the appearance of cellulite on your skin. Cellulite is more noticeable when your skin loses elasticity and thins. Collagen aids in retaining more moisture within your skin, and smooths out wrinkles.

#3 - Strengthens, Repairs and Strengthens hair and Nails

As you age and ages, issues like fall hair and brittle nails are more apparent. Hair can also become dry and thin, and nails could break or breaking off. The reason for this is that the body begins to lose collagen protein which is vital for healthy nails and hair. Recent studies suggest that collagen may reverse the loss of hair.

#4 Repairs To A Leaky Gut Gut

Around 60-80% of our immune system is located within the gut. Leaky gut is the most frequent reason for thyroid dysfunction and an autoimmune disorder. If someone suffers from leaky gut, toxins, infections and other toxins. could pass through their intestinal wall, and then enter the bloodstream. This can cause inflammation that may, in time, cause autoimmune disorders. The amino acids that make collagen stop the leakage by actively creating new tissue, and also healing damaged cells.

#5 - Helps Improve Sleep

There's nothing more beneficial to the human body as a restful night's rest. It's essential to an energised mind and body. Eight hours of sleep can help you look healthier, boosts your concentration, boosts your mood and may even help you shed weight.

However, with the demands of modern life sleep is often the only thing at the bottom of the priority list. As a result, fatigue can take its toll. Collagen aids in falling asleep quicker and enjoy a more restful sleep. Contrary to sleep aids which can cause you to feel sleepy the next day.

#6 - Helps Maintain Hormonal Balance

Research has shown that amino acids found in collagen may help maintain the balance of amino acids within the body. They also assist in hormone production.

#7 - Improves Digestion

Collagen assists to heal the intestinal tract and repair the mucous liner. It helps improve digestion by breaking down proteins and fats from food. Consuming collagen peptides prior to meals can boost the absorption of proteins within your body.

#8 - Aids in Weight Management

Glycine, an amino acid that is found in collagen, is a key ingredient in building muscles that are lean. Because muscle burns higher calories than fat, having a leaner muscles boosts your metabolism. Even when you're not working collagen can help your body's body burn more calories and helps to keep your weight under control. There are studies that suggest collagen can reduce appetite.

#9 - Detoxifies Your Liver

Everyday we are exposed tons of toxic substances. It's difficult to figure out what to do to reverse their effects on our bodies. This is why a detox every day is essential. It helps reduce the negative effects of toxins that are present in the body. A small dose of collagen in your breakfast each day is a fantastic method to cleanse the liver.

The amino acids that make up collagen "glycine" aids in the reduction of the risk of liver damage. It also helps in the rapid elimination of the liver which is the reason a lot of people make bone broth a regular part in their daily diet.

#10 - Promotes healthy teeth and Gums

The collagen not only helps to create the structure of teeth, it also strengthens the tissues surrounding teeth. Contrary to braces, surgeries, and tooth-whitening products it works on the inside to ensure you maintain beautiful and healthy teeth. Collagen gives you the nutrients that your mouth health wouldn't obtain.

Collagen Cream

Each year, hundreds of collagen creams are introduced into the market. They are often considered to be the next big thing in anti-aging creams. In most instances, there's more advertising behind them than actual science.

There are a small number of substances that are capable of reproducing collagen and they all require the proper quantity to function.

Many creams for anti-wrinkle available currently contain a collagen-building mechanism, but the quantity can differ based on the formulation. The active ingredients contained in these formulations could increase collagen production and smooth wrinklesand fine lines, etc.

However, applying collagen-based formulas on your skin might not be as beneficial as you believe, since the skin isn't absorption of the collagen. The collagen molecules aren't so small as they have to be to fully absorb into the skin.

Collagen injections can be extremely efficient but they last just a few months. Injectables on the other on the other hand, can alter facial contours, resulting in an unnatural appearance. The chance of having side negative effects or physical discomfort are always present with these choices. Additionally, they're costly and require a physician's appointment.

Collagen Pills

Collagen supplements have long been considered by some to be the ultimate anti-aging potion for skin. A study has found that taking collagen supplements may help joints and bones by providing the body with a bio-available source of amino acids.

Collagen pills usually contain as much as one milligram of collagen in each pill. They can mix different kinds of collagen and Vitamin C. This increases your body's production of collagen. Vitamin C is an important component in the production of collagen within the body. According to research published in American Journal of Clinical Nutrition A higher concentration of vitamin C is linked with a lesser risk of the appearance of wrinkles.

Because the hydrolysed Collagen has a intense after-taste when consumed as its own, sugaror other sweeteners or juices are commonly added to the formula. This is why it's crucial to pay attention to the sugar content within your collagen capsules or tablets. Sometimesthe ingredient that sweetens will not be identified on the label. It happens because certain brands are made with the high-fructose corn syrup which is the most affordable type of sugar source.

Another ingredient to be taken note of can be artificial sugar. They can lead to long-term health problems. A study published in Journal of Toxicology and Environmental Health, Critical Reviews, indicates that Sucralose is an artificial sugar may cause a range of negative biological issues within the body. Sucralose is commonly used by collagen supplement makers.

People who are having difficulty taking collagen pills can explore other collagen supplements such as liquid and powder.

Let's proceed to our next chapter, which is about foods that boost collagen.

Chapter 3: Diets That Boost Collagen

"The future doctor will not be around anymore."
treat the human frame using medications,
Instead, it will treat and prevent illness through nutrition."
-- Thomas Edison

The body is constantly replenishing collagen levels to repair damaged but it isn't able to do the same thing for a long time. As collagen production within the body starts to decrease and the quality of collagen begins to decrease as well. This is when the body requires constant supply of collagen via supplements, products for the skin and foods.

The right diet is crucial to boost the collagen production in your body. As we all know, prevention is better than treatment, which is why eating a diet that is with a low sugar content and a high in colorful fruits and vegetables is highly advised.

Here are the top foods that boost collagen.

Avocados

Avocados and avocado oil are rich in omega-3 which helps to boost collagen. Additionally, they contain vitamin E that fights free radicals within the bloodstream Similar to Matcha tea.

Fish

Tuna and salmon are high in omega-3 fatty acids, which strengthens cells according to nutritionist from New York Brook Alpert. The stronger cells can aid in skin health.

Organic Lean Protein

Similar to our muscles like our muscles, collagen needs protein to increase strength. Other than fish, excellent sources of organic lean protein are nuts or lean meat, as well as egg whites. Egg whites are a great source of proline as well as lysine that are vital in the process of building collagen.

Dark Green Vegetables

The greens of Kale and spinach are rich in antioxidants. They are also similar to Matcha tea. Like Matcha tea the greens offer protection from free radicals that are present in the blood.

Red Vegetables

Red fruits and vegetables like beets tomatoes, and red peppers are high in lycopene. It boosts collagen levels in the body. It also helps keep your skin safe from sun-induced damage.

Orange Vegetables

Orange vegetables such as sweet potatoes and carrots have lots of vitamin A that helps repair damaged collagen.

Garlic

Garlic contains lipoic acid as well as taurine, which are two active ingredients that help rebuild collagen. It's also a good source of sulphurthat is a key ingredient in the production of collagen.

Berries

Blackberries and raspberries contain phytonutrients that aid collagen fibres join in a manner that aids the body in producing more collagen.

Chocolate

Dark chocolate baking is abundant in zinc, a mineral which repairs damaged cells, decreases inflammation and boosts collagen production. Zinc is also a protector of the collagen as well as elastin. Other foods that are rich in zinc include oysters, white mushrooms as well as flax seeds, pumpkin seeds wheat germ, squash seeds etc.

Citrus Fruits

Numerous studies have suggested that citrus fruits such as citrus fruits like lime, lemon, and grapefruit could aid with two essential amino acids, which are lysine as well as proline, transform into collagen with ease. They are high in vitamin C, which is vital in neutralising free radicals as well as preventing collagen from breaking down.

Soya

Sources like soyamilk as well as cheese, tofu and tofu contain plant hormones that act as antioxidants and boost collagen production. They also aid in aiding the skin in blocking the skin-aging enzymes.

Matcha Green Tea

As the most concentrated type of green tea Matcha is a rich source of polyphenols. These shield the surface against UV damage. Both UVA light as well as UVB light damage the skin, by penetrating various layers of the skin. They could result in DNA destruction, lower the levels of antioxidant enzymes, cause an oxidative stress, trigger inflammation and can cause the birth of tumours and accelerate the ageing process on the face.

Matcha green tea helps protect skin fibroblasts from dying. This is a thorough report on how Matcha aids in fighting the signs of ageing on your skin.

Bone Broth and Collagen

Bone broths like fish, chicken, beef lamb and others are a staple in traditional diets throughout the world. They are the foundation of fine food. Their reason is that they are high in nutrients, easy to digest, uncomplicated, and are bursting with flavor.

Bones and marrow, tendon and ligaments, feet and skin are the body parts of an animal that cannot be eaten in a single bite, but their benefits to health can be absorbed into your body through simmering them for some days and drinking the broth.

If simmered, ligaments and bones release healing compounds like glutamine, proline and collagen. They can make you healthier.

Two researchers in nutrition from the Weston A. Price Foundation, Sally Fallon and Kaayla Daniel, have revealed the fact that bone broth is rich in minerals. The minerals inside bone broth and are present in a readily digestible form. In addition bone broth also has calcium silicon, magnesium and phosphorus. It also contains sulphur, as well as chondroitin sulphate and glucosamine. These two compounds are utilized in supplements to help reduce arthritis pain and swelling, and arthritis.

Bone broth is an excellent source of all amino acids your body requires, as well as gelatin, collagen trace minerals, numerous other nutrients that aren't readily available from other, often found food items that we consume daily.

What is the reason why some people are adding Collagen to Coffee?

Coffee in the morning can be a common habit for many. The research suggests that coffee could provide several benefits for health. Incorporating collagen peptides into coffee boosts these benefits and improves overall health.

In addition to providing the energy needed to get going, this supplement also balances the caffeine rush with protein. It means it is possible to stay active for a prolonged time, and also have a healthier body.

Incorporating a tablespoon of collagen peptides into your morning coffee is easy and much faster than waiting hours for bone broth ready to cook. The same health benefits of bone broth.

When it is added to coffee it's not a big difference in flavour, taste or texture, as collagen is flavorless and smellless. It disintegrates quickly into liquids, but it tends to create gelatinous clumps with an appearance similar to pearls of tapioca found in bubble tea. They also taste similar to yeast. It doesn't leave a lingering taste that means it can be enjoyed alongside other food items.

Consuming coffee that is rich in collagen has become an increasingly popular choice for famous and well-known celebrities like actresses Jennifer Aniston and Busy Philipps and fashion designer Tamara Mellon, Bulletproof Coffee founder and biohacking businessman Dave Asprey, and a variety of well-known health bloggers. In addition to coffee, some include collagen in their smoothies and shakes after a workout.

One of the most common concerns about collagen among mothers who are expecting is whether it's safe to use collaxin during the pregnancy. This topic will be discussed in the next chapter.

Chapter 4: It Safe To Take Collagen While Pregnant?

"The time a baby is born, their mother also gets born.

She was never present prior to. The woman was there but the mother never.

A mother is absolutely brand new."

Osho

A common concern for expecting mothers concerns whether collagen supplementation during pregnancy is secure. There are many advantages to collagen supplements, and, if you're pregnant these benefits may be even more crucial for your health as well as your baby's.

Collagen is basically protein and protein is essential to the well-being and health of women in the midst of pregnancy. The quantity of proteins consumed throughout pregnancy may influence the baby's weight and body composition, as well as head circumference and could cause chronic health issues like cardiovascular diseases, diabetes and overweight.

Mothers who don't eat sufficient protein during pregnancy may be at the risk of having premature births. But a diet that is high in protein may result in other problems. So, a healthy balance has to be kept.

Women who are pregnant constantly use their bodies to help carry the burden of their newborn babies. Their bodies are under many strains and energy is depleted during pregnancy. If they don't have sufficient nutrients and their bodies begin to get energy from their internal stores of minerals and vitamins. These minerals and vitamins reside in bones, and if they are taken in by the body in order to supply nutrients to the baby during the womb, this could cause harm to the mother's overall health since these minerals and vitamins are essential to the total body.

If there's not enough collagen in bones, their structure loses the strength needed for calcification to take place. The bones will require hydrolysed collagen because it is the most crucial protein that supports joint health. Two amino acids present in the hydrolysed collagen such as proline and glycine, help in the three-dimensional conformation of collagen. They also help maintain the stability of cartilage collagen.

Collagen is the protein that helps in the buoyancy of the pregnant woman's body. It does not just aid in maintaining the skin's elasticity, but helps to provide a more peaceful sleep and is among the most essential aspects a woman during pregnancy needs for herself and her baby. The glycine found in collagen helps promote better sleep by keeping an edgier core temperature while the body is resting. It won't aid in falling to sleep faster however, once you're asleep, it aids the body get in the deep sleep state for a prolonged period. It also decreases the sleepiness of the day.

When you are considering taking any supplement however, it is suggested to consult your physician. Your doctor will guide you the best amount of protein you require during pregnancy and the type of protein you should be taking according to your medical background.

Let's look at the nutritional facts of collagen in our next chapter.

Chapter 5: Collagen Nutrition Facts

"These little items - nutrition, location
temperature, recreation
the entire saga of selfishness more
significant
over everything that one has believed to
be important to date."
Friedrich Nietzsche

Collagen is abundant in minerals like
manganese, copper and vitamin C. It is
most well-known as a protein rich in
nutrients that which the body requires in
large quantities. This is due in part to the
number of different kinds of amino acids
in collagen, such as essential conditions,
non-essential, and conditional.

Contrary to what they say the non-
essential amino acids are extremely
crucial. Although the body produces them
under normal conditions but it's not able
to make the amino acids in moments of
stress, illness and other such. When these
conditions arise the body requires
assistance by external sources, such as
supplements and food.

Collagen is an excellent source of amino acids that are not essential like proline, glycine glutamine, arginine, and glutamine. Proline isn't present in abundance in animal flesh, but in sources such as organ meats. The people who don't eat organ meats are suffering from a shortage in these amino acids.

Collagen is composed of a significant amount of hydroxyproline as well as hydroxylysine. As per the George Mateljan Foundation, foods that contain these amino acids may contribute to the production and maintenance of collagen. They are most commonly found on egg whites, and in wheat germ as well as other plant and animal-based food sources.

Vitamin C is the key ingredient that transforms those two amino acids to usable collagen. Bone health and collagen production is dependent on the quantity of Vitamin C in your diet. Vitamin C protects collagen from the damage from free radicals. The most potent vitamins C include papaya, citrus fruits, strawberries, broccoli and bell peppers.

The Phytonutrients play a significant role in the breakdown of collagen. The phytonutrients in green tea have been proven to provide our bodies with vitamins to protect collagen structures.

The dark-colored fruits and berries are also excellent sources of collagen-building nutrients. Sources of phytonutrients from fruits include blueberries and cranberries as well as raspberries and cherries.

Discussions about the benefits of collagen is not complete without a discussion of the information about the nutritional value of collagen in bone broth. Therefore, let's begin by making homemade bone broth.

5.1. The nutritional information for homemade bone broth

Quantity Per 100 grams

Calories - 267

Total Fat 14 g 21 percent

Fat saturated - 3.4 grams 17 percent

The polyunsaturated fat is 4.5 grams

Monounsaturated fat 5 g

Cholesterol 13 mg - 4 3

Sodium - 23,875 mg 994%

Potassium - 309 mg 8%

Total Carbohydrate - 18g 6 %
Dietary fibre - 0g 100 percent
Sugar - 17 g
Protein - 17 g34%
Vitamin A - 0%Vitamin C - 1%
Calcium - 18% Iron - 5%
Vitamin D - 0%Vitamin B-6 - 5%
Vitamin B-12 - 5% Magnesium - 14 percent
Information about the nutritional content of tablets of collagen:
Amount Per Serving
Calories33Sodium28 mg
The Total Fat2 GPotassium 0 mg
Saturated1 gTotal Carbs0 G
Polyunsaturated0 gDietary Fiber0 g
Monounsaturated0gSugars0g
Trans0 gProtein4 g
Cholesterol0 mg
Vitamin A0%Calcium0%
Vitamin C0%Iron0 percent

The nutritional facts of collagen pills:
Amount Per Serving
Calories412Sodium135 mg
The Total Fat16 grams of Potassium 0 mg

Satinated11 gTotal Carbs62 g

Polyunsaturated0 gDietary Fiber0 g

Monounsaturated0gSugars0g

Trans1 gProtein5 g

Cholesterol0 mg

Vitamin A0%Calcium0%

Vitamin C 0%Iron 0 The percentage

Collagen drinks have nutritional facts:

Amount Per Serving (125 milliliters)

Calories65Sodium0 mg

The Total Fat0 is gPotassium0 milligrams

Saturated0 gTotal Carbs6 grams

Polyunsaturated0gDietary Fibre0g

Monounsaturated0 gSugars0

Trans0 gProtein10 g

Cholesterol0 mg

Vitamin A0%Calcium0%

Vitamin C 0%Iron 0 In %

Collagen powder nutrition facts:

Quantity Per Serving (1 tablespoon)

Calories30Sodium0 mg

The Total Fat0 is a gPotassium 0 mg

Saturated0 GTotal Carbs3 g

Polyunsaturated0 gDietary Fiber0 g

Monounsaturated0 gSugars0

Trans0 gProtein8 g

Cholesterol0 mg

Vitamin A0%Calcium0%

Vitamin C0%Iron0 percent

It is a good idea to supply your body with nutrients by consuming collagen sources such as fish, beef, and eggs, or supplements made of these. Next chapter we'll look at these collagen sources.

Chapter 6: Compared: Bovine, Chicken And Marine Collagen

"Our food is our medicine, and

Our medicine should be in the food we eat."

Hippocrates

Collagen comes from mammals from all over the animal kingdom. It is extracted out of the skin and tendons. Collagen is classified into three types kinds, including:

Type I is a result of the tendons

Type I as well as Type III are skin conditions that result from the skin

Type II is derived from cartilage

The majority of collagen supplements are taken from chickens, cows and pigs as well as fish. Bovine collagen has the ability to directly increase the production of collagen within the body.

Chicken collagen is believed to be beneficial in supporting cartilage within the body. This is why collagen supplements of type II collagen supplements are made from chicken.

Marine collagen can be found in the scales of fish or skin, which is typically made from cold-water fish such as salmon.

The scales typically contain more collagen protein. They also tend to be more nutritious. value.

Bioavailability

Marine collagen is absorbed much more easily in the body because it has a higher bioavailability over bovine collagen. The reason for this is due to the fact that marine collagen has smaller particles when compared to other forms of collagen. Because of the smaller dimensions, particles facilitates the absorption of collagen peptides in the skin, as well as other parts like joints and bones. This aids in the creation of collagen. Because collagen is absorbed into skin in such a way it is thought to be the most effective source of collagen for skin. Chicken collagen is the most well-known collagen ingredient used frequently in medical practice.

Price-wise

Bovine collagen is more affordable to extract, and that is why it is utilized in a variety of cosmetic products. This is by far the most sought-after kind of collagen supplement available there. But, up to 3percent of people are thought to have an allergy to bovine collagen.

The body's reaction

The body may respond to the peptide chains in bovine collagen. This can cause a severe allergic reaction. But marine collagen contains less apparent antigens and more suitable peptide chains, which minimizes the possibility of allergic reactions. This is the reason why marine collagen is believed to be superior to other forms of collagen.

Health benefits in terms of

Bovine collagen benefits:

* Save precious protein - when your blood sugar is at a low level the body may make use of bovine collagen instead burning off its reservoir of muscles.

* Enhances sleep. When taken prior to bedtime collagen's glycine can increase

the quality of sleep and may even decrease fatigue in the daytime.

* Accelerates the healing process of wounds Collagen combats bacteria that cause the wounds. The wounds remain sterile, and assists in speedier healing of wounds. A study has found that collagen hydrolysing from beef will speed up the healing process of ulcers by 200%..

Improves the gut health * Improves the health of your gut Collagen can have a healing and gentle effect on the gastrointestinal tract. It improves stomach acid levels , which could boost digestive health and the function of your gut.
Chicken collagen benefits:
* Relief from arthritis - Chicken collagen is a rich source of joint-healthy chondroitinsulfate as well as an ingredient called glucosamine, which provides relief from osteoarthritis as well as arthritis rheumatoid.

* Increases immunity . Research has proven that chicken collagen helps close the openings within the gut's lining. This can improve the immune system.

Improves digestion - Chicken collagen is a great way to maintain the health of the mucous layer within the digestive tract. This prevents leaky gut syndrome that is typically the root cause of food allergies, autoimmune diseases, and other.

* Combats heart disease - Certain studies suggest that chicken collagen can help fight heart disease. Due to its inflammation-fighting ability, it could be used to reduce the risk of heart disease.
Marine collagen benefits:
* Gives skin an attractive glow Marine collagen is a hugely sought-after ingredient in the beauty world due to its capacity to increase collagen production within the skin.

* Starts working faster as other forms of collagen. Marine collagen contains fewer

protein peptides, which make it more easily absorbed by the surface of your skin, than bovine or chicken collagen. Due to its easy absorption, the synthesis of marine collagen begins to occur quicker than other collagen types.

* Includes 8 of the nine essential amino acids. amino acids found in marine collagen perform a variety of important functions within the body, like building muscle mass and lean mass, stopping the formation in stomach ulcers and increasing the tolerance of glucose, thereby helping to prevent diabetes, and preventing cell damage , etc.

Reduces levels of cholesterol In clinical studies marine collagen was shown to reduce LDL cholesterol (bad cholesterol) and to increase HDL (good cholesterol). It's also believed to assist in regulating the in regulating the metabolism of lipids.

More of a comparison

Marine collagen is the type I collagen, while bovine collagen is of type II or III. Marine collagen is lower in the amount of hydroxyproline that gives it an lower temperature of denaturation. The lower content of hydroxyproline helps your body's digestive system to absorb, compared with bovine collagen.

Odor is a concern with collagen. Bovine collagen is generally stinky when it is present at 33%. Marine collagen is, however isn't as bad and is able to be tolerated until the concentration is around 10 percent.

In addition, excessive consumption of bovine collagen can make our bodies store bovine collagen with the fat it comes with. This isn't the situation with marine collagen, which is not retained in our bodies and, in addition, is smaller in fat content when in comparison to bovine collagen.

The content of hydroxyproline of chicken collagen lower than bovine collagen. Aspartic and glutamic acid residues found in chicken collagen may be similar to skin of calf collagen.

Once you are aware of the various collagen types as well as their advantages and distinctions to make informed choices about which one is right for you. Let's look at how collagen aids in fat loss and weight reduction in the following chapter.

Chapter 7: Collagen For Weight Loss

"Great things don't happen on impulse, but rather by

A collection of little objects arranged."

Vincent Van Gogh

Collagen supplements are being increasingly utilized to lose weight and improving overall health. There are numerous positive effects that collagen supplements can have on weight loss. For example, hydrolysed collagen can be utilized to act as an ingredient active in a variety of weight loss supplements, specifically those that are available in liquid form. They are considered to be beneficial during sleep.

As per Brigham and Women's Hospital, Hydrolysed collagen can also be believed to be a treatment for joint pain from arthritis. In addition, certain people believe that collagen will improve muscle mass and lean mass with the body's fat-burning process.

There are a lot of claims that have been proven and unproven there is one question to be asked: can collagen actually help you shed weight? Let's see if we can answer this.

There are a lot of reasons to agree that collagen does have some weight loss effects. First it is important to consider the fact that collagen plays a crucial part in the growth of muscle. Because it promotes growth in muscle mass it is reasonable to believe that growth will exhaust the energy stored within the body. This will result in fat loss.

The increase in muscle mass has an immediate impact in the quantity of calories consumed every day by the body. It also leads to the body losing more weight and assists in the process of metabolism.

Reshaping your figure is an advantage that collagen supplements claim to provide. This is due to collagen's capacity to keep skin and muscles firm and plump. The decreased appetite that may result from a consistent intake of collagen can result in an overall more toned, firmer appearance. Consuming collagen on a regular basis can benefit those who are prone to eating too much.

Certain studies have indicated that collagen peptides are 40% more satisfying than other proteins and help people feel "full" quicker. There are studies that also suggest that collagen could induce our body's production of "satiating" hormones.

But, despite these assertions, there isn't any tangible evidence to prove that collagen does indeed aid with weight reduction.

Additionally, because the hydrolysed collagen ingredient is bovine or marine cartilage or bones it cannot be used by vegans, vegetarians and people who are allergic to shellfish.

Collagen and Cellulite

Once you've figured out the ways collagen can assist in weight loss, you might think about the issue of cellulite, which is usually related to weight issues.

Collagen peptide supplements can aid in shedding the cellulite, and also shape the body in general. Cellulite usually occurs as the result of a deficiency from collagen that is found in dermal areas of skin. The dermal layer of skin holds the fat in the proper position.

How are collagen and cellulite connected

The layer of skin (dermis) is composed of 75 percent collagen, this protein makes up around 90 percent of the total volume of the skin. So, having sufficient collagen is essential to keep the skin's walls the skin smooth and prevent cellulite from forming.

As collagen begins to decrease within the skin, it loses its elasticity and becomes thinner. Cellulite is then apparent. A consistent intake of collagen protein as well as exercising can be extremely beneficial in getting fit, since collagen peptides can boost the amount of energy you have, and heal the fibres the reason for cellulite's appearance.

According to a study collagen supplementation in the diet can reduce appearance of cellulite. The reason for this is because types II and III collagen increase the density of the skin, decreasing its thinness and increasing its elasticity.

Based on the numerous studies completed so far, it appears that collagen is definitely a supplement that may be very beneficial in terms of boosting metabolism in building muscle mass, and decreasing cellulite.

To reap all these benefits, selecting the best collagen supplement is vital. Based on research, here are what to look for when purchasing a collagen supplement:

1. A collagen content greater than eight grams (8000mg)

2. The presence of peptides hydrolysed type I

Like any other medication or food you consume supplements are simply that - it adds to your diet. The increase in collagen levels is an excellent strategy to reduce the appearance of cellulite. But eating enough protein other than exercise and a regular routine is not something to be overlooked.

Collagen and Elastin

The two collagens, elastin and collagen can be found within the body of humans. Each plays a distinct function. They're both abundant in youthful skin, which keeps the skin firm and smooth. As we age, due to the process, the body is producing smaller amounts of the proteins. In addition, UV damage and other causes affect the connective fibers in the skin. Collagen becomes more rigid, leading to the weakening that surrounds the face. The skin becomes thin, stretches and caves, and develops wrinkles. This makes the skin more prone to damage from the environment.

While all the collagen-related changes are happening in the body, it produces less elastin. The existing elastin starts to lose its ability to stretch back. Elastin fibres loose their elasticity and skin begins to lose its shape. The result is noticeable most prominently around the neck, around the eyes and the jaw line.

Why are Collagen and Elastin Always referred to Together?

The terms collagen and elastin are often brought together due to the fact that they both contribute to providing an elastic skin. Because collagen improves the rigidity of skin Elastin allows the skin to stretch before returning to its original form.

Consider collagen as the bodywork or structure of the skin. It gives it strength and provides a foundation. Consider collagen as a substance which is responsible for making certain that your skin regains its original shape after stretching (as when smiling or in various facial movements).

The Difference between Collagen and Elastin

The major advantage of collagen is its strength. It is made up of extremely sturdy fibres and has a large amount of Tensile strength. Elastin is a softening agent that provides and elasticity to skin. It is a crucial component to maintain skin health. It creates a three-dimensional web between collagen fibers.

Elastin is present beyond the skin in different parts such as arteries, lungs and veins. These are the places in which collagen isn't present.

Similarities between Collagen and Elastin

Elastin, like collagen, is an important component in maintaining the youthfulness of the skin. It aids skin tissue increase and decrease in size.

Both collagen and elastic are located in different levels of the dermis. While collagen is found more within the dermis' lower layer, the dermis Elastin is more abundant in the middle layer.

Like collagen the body's production elastin decreases with the passage of time. But, other elements like environmental damage, smoke, stress poor diet, and so on. are also a factor in the content of elastin found in the skin.

Foods that help build Elastin

If you eat a diet that is rich in specific foods, you can aid your body in increasing the levels of elastin. A balanced diet and good nutrition is vital. Below are the foods that are believed to increase elastin levels:

* Guavas
* Bell peppers with red bells
* Strawberries
* Tomatoes
* Watermelon
* Broccoli
* Cauliflower
* Cabbage
* Leafy greens
* Peas
* Beans
* Fortified cereals
* Wheat germ
* Vegetable oil
* Seeds, nuts and nuts
* Bran
* Clover sprouts
* Foods rich in gelatin such as pot roast, aspic, etc.

After you have learned all about the connection with collagen, weight loss as well as cellulite and collagen, as well as collagen and elastin we'll look into treatments for hair loss treatments, lip treatment and injectables in the following chapter.

Chapter 8: Collagen Treatments

"Heart in her mouth, and soul in her eyes,"
As soft as her clime and as sunny like her sky."

Lord Byron

Healthy skin is a plus. As you age, the skin is more flexible and firm. It also has a greater capacity for resiliency. This is due to collagen's strong and strong frame. As we age the skin begins to lose its elasticity. If this is accompanied by things like environmental damage smoking, stress, a poor lifestyle , etc. wrinkles, fine lines, crow's feet , etc. begin to show more clearly.

Unfortunately, as a result of contemporary methods of food processing food preparation, our diets aren't particularly collagen-rich. Additionally factors like excessive sugar levels in foods as well as dehydration and radiation can cause an inevitable decline in collagen production.

Collagen treatments are an excellent method of revitalising the natural collagen in the skin, and to restore your skin's elasticity.

The three most common forms of collagen treatments comprise collagen injections, lip treatment using collagen and hair treatment using collagen.

The treatment options are adapted in accordance with the skin type, age and UV damage on the individual's skin.

Collagen treatment was first applied on patients in the 1970's.

Collagen Injections

Before you decide to undergo collagen injections, it is essential to seek out a reputable doctor. Together, you will discuss the type of results you're hoping to achieve from the procedure. You should also find out how many injections you'll need depending on your medical background. You'll be able to determine the best collagen filler for your needs from this appointment.

If the best filler is chosen it will be a small amount which will be injectable into the outermost part of the skin. This procedure is called skin testing. It's done to find out if you are sensitive to fillers. After the filler has been injected, you'll need to wait for 4 weeks to check the area for signs that indicate an allergy. In the event that there are no reactions to the injection within four weeks you are able to continue by injecting.

The process for injecting collagen secure and easy. Prior to the injection procedure, local anaesthesia will be used to make the area numb. Similar to all medical procedures complications such as redness mild bruising and tenderness may occur around the site of injection.

Collagen is injections into furrows or lines within the skin. Based on the size and extent of wrinkle(s) the number of injections may be required. It takes less than one hour to finish the procedure.

The best patients who can benefit from collagen injections would be who are between the ages of 35 and 60 with smile lines, frown lines , etc.

There are some medical conditions for which collagen injections aren't recommended like:

* Breastfeeding and pregnancy
* Collagen vascular disease
* Autoimmune disease
* Allergies with beef or bovine products.
Allergic reactions to the drug lidocaine.
Speak to your physician if are experiencing some of these. The most effective course of action is to consult experienced cosmetic surgeons, as they will review any medical conditions, analyze any areas that are of concern, and decide on the best treatment to meet your requirements.

Collagen Lip Treatment

As you age, wrinkles begin to appear prominently around the cheekbones and eyes. However, there are other areas just as susceptible to wrinkles those, like lips. The lips aren't immune the aging process and may thus, shrink and diminish in size and.

Collagen fillers may help to preserve the plumpness and fullness of the lips. A lot of wrinkle fillers that attempt to correct crow's feet or marionette lines could be used to enhance the appearance of lips too.

If you're thinking of getting an injection of collagen into your lips make sure you explore the options with your physician.

In recent years collagen injections are now routine to restore the lip plumpness. In the case of collagen fillers, there are two choices - 1. Bovine collagen , and 2. Human collagen.

If it is injected correctly the right way, it's just as efficient as human collagen that is derived using human cells laboratories.

The injections of collagen into the lips can be costly. In addition, there are other expenses to consider like the amount of sessions needed since several sessions are typically needed to get the desired outcomes. But, choosing a low-cost treatment could lead to the possibility of a poor outcome and, can result in a number of adverse negative effects.

Collagen Hair Treatment

Similar to the skin, bones, and muscle, collagen can be also present in hair. Hair is a source of collagen however its capacity to make it starts to decrease as you get older. To address this issue, the collagen hair treatment was developed.

Collagen hair treatment is similar to botox treatments for hair. It's not an chemical treatment. However, it is more concentrated in cleaning. It also lacks hair straightening characteristics. The collagen hair treatment could last as long as three months.

For those who want to maintain the health of their hair, a collagen hair treatments are extremely beneficial.

While DIY options exist however, it is highly recommended that, if you're trying this in the beginning, have it done at an experienced beauty salon. Professionals be able to determine the precise amount of collagen needed to ensure your hair is healthy.

The benefits of Collagen Hair Treatment
Beauty experts believe in these benefits of a collagen hair treatment
* Strengthens hair
* Reduces split ends
* Minimises hair breakage
Smoothens frizzy hair

* Helps protect hair from heat
* Hydrates the scalp
* Prevents dandruff

A treatment for hair loss using collagen is not harmful, however should a person be prone to allergies or reacts to any of the components included in the product to treat the hair the treatment could cause negative side consequences.

If you're aware of collagen injections and treatments Let's learn more about collagen fibres and collagen keratin in the next chapter.

Chapter 9: Collagen Fibres

"Nature provides you with the appearance you'll see at twentyyears old;
It's your job to be worthy of the look you'll get to be able to wear at the age of fifty."
Coco Chanel

Collagen forms fiber meshes that provide durability for the skin. Collagen comprises about 20% of dry skin weight of healthy people. Due to collagen's ability to communicate with itself, as well as different proteins, it assists to strengthen the skin and keep its elasticity.

Collagen is a strong protein that gets its strength from its distinctive protein structure. The amino acid sequence allows it to create a tight, tightly-woven network of fibrils that communicate with each other. The amino acids require a certain degree of modification, which is carried out by enzymes.

Cells like fibroblasts create collagen proteins that are made up of procollagen. After the procollagen has been released by the cell, it's broken down to form active collagen that forms small fibres or fibrils.

Collagen Type I Fibres

Collagen type I creates the triple helix, which consists of 3 chains, or strands. Each one of them contains 10,000 amino acids. Hydrogen bonds between amino acids found in various chains aid them to stay in place. They provide the fiber with a lot of force.

In most cases the multiple collagen triple helices are able to join and create a fibril that is similar to rope that has a high tensile strength.

Collagen Type II Fibres

Collagen types II fibers are less pronounced compared with Collagen types I fibrils. They remain scattered manner within the gelatinous carbohydrate-protein complexes. They link up together with the collagen type IX. Due to its structure collagen type IX does not create fibrils in the same way that other collagen types do, however, it is able to keep fibers of collagen II in place.

Collagen type II fibrils give cartilage with the strength and elasticity it requires.

Collagen Type III Fibres

Although collagen type III doesn't possess the same strength as Type I, but it also forms triple helices, with great endurance. Collagen kind III is typically located in the intestines, blood vessels, and even in the skin. Since it is produced faster that type I, our body makes it quickly when skin is damaged for example, as it is in the case of a wound.

The decomposition of collagen fibers can be a major benefit that can be derived by body massage. Massages that are effective for the body help collagen fibres to align to reduce pain, increases relaxation and decreases restrictions in movement of the body.

The decomposition and realignment of collagen fibers can be extremely useful in these circumstances:

* Post-surgery
* Post injury
* Scarring

There are numerous benefits to collagen degrading and realigning such as the reduction in scar tissue better recovery, and a greater flexibility.

A variety of methods like kneading and frictions are employed to get the desired results.

Collagen and Keratin

Keratin is an elastic structural protein present in all animals and can be found in various places like hair nail, skin hair, horns, etc.

Keratin is also made from multiple amino acids that bind together in sheets that are joined through hydrogen bonds.

Keratin is just as sturdy as collagen, it's but not as helical.

The collagen as well as keratin can be described as highly insoluble and have a high tension strength. But their structures are distinct, due to the distinct tasks they fulfill.

The fibrous proteins are typically long. Keratin is not an exception. Keratin hair strands are quite long.

Keratin treatment for smoothness, which are similar as the collagen treatment, have become incredibly well-known. They are able to help you get rid of hair that is frizzy and help it become more manageable. The treatments are essentially replenishing the hair's protein loss with a formulation that is made up of Keratin, along with other ingredients.

Keratin treatments take around 90 minutes or more according to the length of hair. Results differ based on the type of hair and the nature of the treatment. For collagen treatments, it is recommended that you have it done by a professional at the salon since they be the best at using Keratin to minimize the damage to hair.

Keratin treatments can give your hair a luster but it's not an absolute. For the best results, it's recommended to undergo the treatment every four months.

Because it's an chemical process, it could result in allergic reactions. Thus, those who have sensitive scalps must be extra cautious. It is recommended to speak with an experienced dermatologist before deciding to undergo this treatment.

The next chapter will discuss the hydrolysed collagen and collagen Hyaluronic Acid.

Chapter 10: Hydrolysed Dissolved

Collagen As Well As Hyaluronic Acid

"There there is more knowledge to your body
rather than in your most profound philosophy."
Friedrich Nietzsche

Hydrolyzed Collagen is a type of collagen, which can be called by various other names like collagen peptides, collagen hydrolysate gelatine, hydrolysed gelatine collagen hydrolysate gelatine hydrolysate and peptides hydrolysed by collagen.

It's composed of tiny amino acids that aid in the creation of collagen that is created in the body. Some claim it could boost the lean muscle mass stores as well as treat arthritis and even strengthen specific organs.

Hydrolysed collagen is extracted from bovine bone and cartilage. The process for obtaining this involves crushing and grinding of bone. Then, they soak the bones in acid to eliminate calcium. Then, it is re-soaked to break collagen bonds, and then drying. The collagen is derived from the tissues beneath cow hides.

It is a distinct amino acid profile that mostly consists of glycine glutamic acid and proline as well as the amino acid alanine. Amino acids get swiftly taken up into bloodstreams. The body uses them as building blocks for the creation of new collagen.

Utilization and health benefits

Hydrolysed collagen is rapidly gaining recognition as a protein substitute. In the medical sector, it's employed in post-surgery treatments such as joint sore recovery, and cancer recovery treatments. In weight loss programs it is utilized as a fantastic alternative to standard meals since it aids in maintaining glucose levels increasing energy levels and providing the body with amino acids. It can also be utilized as a coating for capsules for various medications.

Hydrolysed collagen can be helpful in joint pain relief as well as muscles pain relief. It also increases the body's production of protein and aids in the growth of muscles mass.

Clinical studies have proven that supplements with hydrolysed collagen aid athletes suffering from joint pain. It also helps reduce the risk of joint damage.

Hyaluronic Acid

Hyaluronic acid is a naturally occurring glycosaminoglycan. This is it is a type of polysaccharide that is an essential component in connective tissue. It is derived from a variety of sources, including food, supplements, and supplements. The epithelial, connective and neural tissue, it is responsible for several important organs within the body.

As with collagen, hyaluronic Acid is produced naturally by the body in various areas, such as eyes sockets in joints, on the skin, etc. It's a clearand oily substance that helps keep collagen, improve moisture levels and increase elasticity as well as flexibility.

The average human body has about 15g of hyaluronic acids and synthesizes about one third of it each day.

Benefits

Hyaluronic acid aids in the function of soft tissues, like joint support. It assists in the fight against osteoarthritis, and is a part of the reason for the development of cartilage's strength.

Its unique capacity to hold in moisture and to adjust the rate of absorption in accordance with the fluctuating levels of humidity within the atmosphere, hyaluronic acid has an vital role in maintaining the health of your skin.

It also shields the surface against UVA and UVB Rays.

If taken as an oral supplement it plays an important part in collagen production. It aids the body to produce collagen at its normal rate.

Similarities to Collagen

Both collagen and hyaluronic acid are organic compounds that occur in connective tissues throughout the body.

The results of research have shown that both are able to slow down some of the signs that are physical aging like wrinkles and lines Crow's feet, etc. and improve the skin's tone.

The Difference between Collagen as well Hyaluronic Acid

Collagen is fibrous protein. In contrast, hyaluronic acids is a kind of polysaccharide. Collagen

is present in cartilage, bones, connective tissues, the fibres that runs through the skin as well as tendon. The hyaluronic acid located in the deeper layers of the skin , referred to as"the "Dermis".

Collagen's primary function is to give the strength, resilience and elasticity. Hyaluronic acid's primary purpose is to cushion and lubrication for tissues and joints.

Hydrolysed collagen as well as the hyaluronic acids can reduce the appearance of wrinkles, age spots, and improve joint health. It is sensible to supplement these with supplements for well-being and healthy joints as well as beautiful skin. But, it's best to consult with your doctor prior to beginning taking these supplements.

In the next section, we will discuss vegan collagen and the possibility of being able to obtain it.

Chapter 11: Can You Get Vegan Collagen?

"Animals have come to us and are and not to be a threat to us."

- Anonymous

If you're a vegan, you are aware that it can be difficult to find vegan alternatives for food that typically is derived from animals.

Collagen is not vegan or vegetarian.

Is it possible to obtain it from plants?

The majority of commercially available collagen-based products originate from animal sources. But, if we provide our bodies with the ingredients needed to make collagen, for example, nutritious natural foods, we can assist our bodies create the collagen that we require to remain healthy and youthful.

It's true that there is no need to consume animal products for your collagen needs. Other than topical vegan items There are some foods that can be incorporated into your diet to boost the body's natural collagen production.

The following are the best vegan options for a natural collagen booster.

Silica

As collagen is the primary ingredient of beautiful hair, beautiful skin as well as nails, silica also is also the element that makes collagen. Silica from plants contains more than animals, making it a fantastic option for vegetarians and vegans. The best Silica source is commonly known as the horsetail (Equisetum arvense) stem. Contrary to what its name suggests it's a plant that absorbs silicon from soil.

Nature-based Sources for Hyaluronic Acid

The most effective naturally-sourced source for hyaluronic acids is seaweeds, such as Kelp. However, soya-based products like mango, avocados and sweet potatoes are also good sources.

White Tea

Based on a study carried out in Kingston University, white tea may help protect the skin's structural proteins and collagen, particularly. It's believed that it can block the activity of enzymes that break down collagen, which causes wrinkles and fine lines.

Black and green Olives
Sulphur-rich foods have a significant role to play in increasing collagen production in the body. Green and black olives are high in sulfur. Apart from helping collagen production, they reduce oil production as well, which is a great benefit for people with acne-prone or oily skin.

Avocado Oil
Avocado oil is in use for some time, and has been proven scientifically to possess the capacity to stimulate your body to make more collagen. The oil is high in plant steroids, and easily accessible to the system, the avocado oil could effectively minimize the appearance of acne or age spots. It can be applied topically and also added to your diet. It is also possible to add more avocados into your diet for the maximum benefits.

Almonds
Almonds are a great food for your skin. They're a great source of protein that

stimulates collagen production. They're also high in healthy monounsaturated fatty acids along with vitamin B1, B5, and B6 and copper, calcium, magnesium, zinc along with Vitamin E. Magnesium is a great mineral for your nervous systemand gives you relief for your skin from effects of anxiety and stress. In turn the appearance of wrinkles and fine lines reduces.

But, it's more beneficial to eat raw almonds or sprouted raw almonds instead of the roasted varieties. Almond butter made from raw almonds is an excellent option , too.

Seeds and Nuts

Chia seeds and pumpkin seeds hemp seeds, sunflower seeds, flax seeds chestnuts, coconut Pecans, Pistachios, Pistachios, and cashews are high in compounds that aid your body's natural production of collagen.

Tahini

Tahini is another term used to describe Sesame Seed Butter. It's an extremely efficient food for your skin because it is rich in calcium zinc vitamin B1 iron as well as protein. Vitamin B1 helps to prevent thiamin deficiencies and helps your skin improve its health, giving you the strength you need and protecting your body from fatigue. Tahini also contains copper which minimizes fine lines, aids in collagen production and lessens inflammation. It is best to use uncooked Tahini.

You'll Need A Lot Of Vitamin C To Collagen Keep in mind that there is no collagen without vitamin C.

The collagen-making process gets impaired, and this can lead to a variety of health issues. Vitamin C insufficiently affects the ability of bones to create collagen. When collagen is broken down and isn't replaced, joints begin to wear out, and the tendons begin to shrink. The whole body begins to fall apart.

As humans do not have the capacity to create vitamin C on their own, food and supplements to diets are essential for supplying vitamin C. And the best part is that the most potent Vitamin C sources are plants.

Include plenty of citrus fruit, Kale broccoli, red peppers and rose hips into your diet to ensure you have enough vitamin C. The extract of rosehips itself is high with collagen. This means that including it in your diet can be beneficial.

Let's discuss collagen oil later in the following chapter.

Collagen Oil

"I'm an avid believer that, if you concentrate on great skincare,

You really don't require much make-up."

Demi Moore

For products that are applied to the skin like creams and lotions with collagen collagen molecules are too big to be absorbed by the skin. However, there are many other ways to naturally increase the production of collagen in your body to benefit your skin. Utilizing essential oils in certain ways is just one of them.

Its molecular weight is tiny and helps the skin absorb them effectively. Essential oils possess beneficial properties that nourish the skin which makes it soft and smooth. Essential oils are beneficial in boosting collagen production.

Massage therapists rub oil into the skin, they typically dilute essential oils by using an oil carrier like almond oil or olive oil. This is due to the fact that essential oils are a concentrated extract of the plants they are made from. When applied to skin, without diluting, the concentrated extract of plants within them could cause harm.

The Most Effective Collagen Oil

The most effective oil for promoting collagen production within the human body would be avocado oil. It is, however, intended for use internally and not applied topically.

According to a study in 2006 released in Journal of Rheumatology, avocado oil is a powerful source of the type II collagen.

Avocado oil is not only extremely beneficial in smoothing and hydrating the skin, it's widely recommended for its effectiveness as the best approach to treat acne, blackheads and other forms of skin irritation. Additionally, it's known for its ability to diminish wrinkles, age spots and wrinkles.

Replace your olive oil using avocado oil for salad dressings, and similar dishes can be a lot of benefits for your skin.

Cold-pressed avocado oil is among the top sources of monounsaturated fat acids such as Oleic acid. These fatty acids are an excellent addition to your diet , but they also can influence the appearance and feel on your face.

But be aware that results for each individual may differ in accordance with the type of skin and other variables like the diet, lifestyle, etc.

It is crucial to look for cold-pressed, unrefined avocado oil as it is rich in restorative qualities for the skin that refined avocado oil lacks. Cold-pressed avocado oil is subjected to an extremely minimal refinement process that retains the sterols and chlorophyll as well as vitamin E and antioxidants contained in the oil. It is no surprise that these ingredients are excellent for the skin.

Other oils that you can Make Use of

Here are ten essential oils that start the chain reaction that improves skin elasticity.

1. Lemon Essential Oil

Lemon oil is a hefty amount of vitamin C making it an excellent collagen-boosting oil. It's also one of the most readily accessible essential oil in the market.

2. Calendula Essential Oil

Calendula oil is stuffed with flavonoids that stimulate collagen production. Just adding a few drops to the form of a cream for massage and then rubbing it on the skin will enhance the body's ability to produce collagen.

3. Frankincense Essential Oil

In terms of naturally boosting collagen production, the essential oil of frankincense is extremely efficient. Its cytophylactic properties aid in the growth of new cells, while also preventing the existing cells from becoming damaged. It also improves the complexion and tightens and tones wrinkled skin.

4. Carrot Seed Essential Oil

Carrots and their seeds are a source of many antioxidants that heal damaged tissues and build the collagen layer under the skin.

5. Geranium Essential Oil

There are few things that are as beneficial to women's health and wellbeing as geranium essential oil. It aids in resolving menstrual issues regulates hormones, and brings new life to collagen production. It recycles dead cells, and helps the body create new cells.

6. Oil of rosehip

Rosehip oil is rich in Omega 3,6, and 9 in addition to vitamins C, Lycopene, and Linoleic acid. These are extremely potent substances that help in promoting skin cell renewal as well as collagen production. They also reduce wrinkles along with other indicators of aging making the skin soft and moisturized.

7. Sandalwood oil

Sandalwood is renowned for its numerous healing properties. Essential oils of Sandalwood can diminish wrinkles, rejuvenate dull skin, promote healing, and can even function as an anti-inflammatory agent.

8. Eucalyptus oil

Even though it's not yet the most well-known brand in skincare circles, the eucalyptus oils do possess a variety of properties which can improve the condition of skin. It's anti-bacterial as well as anti-microbial, just like tea-tree oils. It aids in treating acne, reduce swelling, redness, and irritation on the skin.

9. Apricot Kernel oil

Apricot Kernel oil has a hefty amount of omega-6 gamma linolenic acid which supplies the skin with vital moisture and nourishment. Vitamin A found helps to promote collagen production and the regeneration and regeneration of the cells on your skin. It's an extremely beneficial oil to heal and moisturize dry skin.

10. Neroli Oil

Essential oil of Neroli is an amazing powerhouse in reducing stretch marks as well as soothing skin. It also helps slow down the process of aging, tightens sagging skin, and smooths wrinkles.

Additionally, the product has a delicate gentle scent.

DIY Collagen Oil Blend Recipe

Make this simple Essential Oil Blend recipe to make an easy DIY fix at home. Take 1 teaspoon of Apricot Kernel Oil, 10 drops of Carrot Seed Essential Oil and 10 drops of Rose Hip Essential Oil and blend them thoroughly. Store the mix within an amber bottle. Use a tiny amount to massage your neck and face following cleansing.

Important points to be aware of:

* Use only 100 percent pure essential oils that are therapeutic grade.

* Prior to applying essential oils, dilute them with an oil carrier (1-3 drops)

* Keep essential oils out from pets and children.

Collagen and Biotin

"I am going to be either 60, or 70 years old and still rocking

My Chanel Blazer with my hair in a coifful way."

Johnny Weir

The last few times have seen an increase in the interest in biotin and collagen for improving hair growth and the quality of hair. This is logical, since collagen and vitamins can be both beneficial to have to do with skin and hair health. Let's examine them, and then shed some light on the extent to which they're efficient.

Although they have distinct roles to perform, biotin and collagen tend to function in a synergistic fashion.

Biotin, also referred to by the name Vitamin B7 and Vitamin H is a B-complex vitamin with water-soluble properties that encourages hair growth and assists in helping eliminate seborrheic skin dermatitis. According to the article entitled "Vitamin H." by The University of Maryland Medical Center.

This vitamin is necessary to promote cell growth within the body, in the process of metabolizing amino acids, fats and other amino acids and the production of fatty acids.

It is often found in foods such as rice, bread whole wheat grains, and leafy green vegetables raw egg yolk chicken, sardines, mushrooms and peanuts Biotin can also be found as an added benefit. However, it is important to be aware that there is no definitive research that indicates that biotin supplements increase the rate of hair growth. Because it is water-soluble any excess can be eliminated by the body in the form of waste.

Collagen increases blood flow in the body. This is important because the healthy growing of hair follicles dependent on a steady flow of blood flow to the follicles. Hair growth is most efficiently when there is an ideal hormone balance within the body. The amino acids contained in collagen aid in maintaining an optimal hormone balance.

The issue is: should you consider supplementing?

Remember Biotin deficiency is very uncommon. So, the fact that you are deficient might not be the case , and it might not be the reason you're having issues in the growth and strength of your hair.

Additionally, biotin cannot stop hair loss. Loss of hair can be caused by either of the two reasons hormone imbalance or genetic causes. Resolving the hormonal imbalances that are present in the body is an ideal alternative to biotin supplements.

If you do decide to take biotin supplements the recommended dose is 2.5mg. Take half of it in your breakfast , and the other half at dinner time over 14 days. When you supplement, you'll require more hydration.

It is suggested that you drink plenty of clean drinking water throughout the day, and eat a balanced diet. The body requires certain vitamins, minerals as well as proteins, fats, and carbohydrates in order to increase the efficacy in biotin supplementation.

There's one negative adverse effect you need to keep in mind. In excess, taking biotin supplements could trigger acne flare-ups. If your skin is susceptible for acne, then it's essential to consult your dermatologist prior to using any supplements.

Do you need to supplement biotin and collagen at simultaneously?

Biotin and collagen are both present in foods and aren't known to interact with one another. But, consulting your physician is recommended.

It's time to learn more about gelatin and collagen. Let's continue to the next section.

Collagen and Gelatin

"The gastric laboratory utilizes its protein ferment

under the influence of an in an acid-reaction."

Ivan Pavlov

Gelatin's story begins with a collagen-like protein. It's the protein that is the most abundantly found in the body. Insufficient levels of it could cause a variety of issues, including eye bags and fine lines to osteoporosis.

Collagen is found in bones and tendons of animal. Think of cuts of beef that have a lot of connective tissues. Cooking turns collagen into gelatin. Gelatin is the cooked form of collagen. Cooking allows us to absorb the amino acids that are beneficial. Gelatin is made up from two amino acids: proline and glycine. These amino acids are essential to maintain good skin but also for nail and hair growth, weight management , and increasing the immune system.

The Unusual Amino Acid Profile of Gelatin

When gelatin is separated from collagen, the gelatin has about 99% of protein in dry weight. Here is what its amino acid composition appears like:

21 percent Glycine

Proline 12%

12 of hydroxyproline

10 percent glutamic acid

9% alanine

8.8 9 % arginamine

Aspartic acid 6%

4 % lysine

Glycine is anti-inflammatory , and research suggests that it may accelerate healing of wounds, enhance sleep quality and make falling asleep more comfortable. A substantial amount of glycine when combined with a balance of amino acids have many benefits for stress relief to provide.

As an added benefit, glycine could be used to aid in recovery from strokes and seizures and also to boost memory. It also increases digestion of acid in the stomach, which improves digestion and the absorption of nutrients.

How Gelatin is Made

The bones, skin and tendons are used to make gelatin.

Our predecessors had better access to these items, since they could use an entire animal for various reasons including cooking dinner or creating bone broth. Bone broth is an incredible way to maximize the benefit of gelatin.

Gelatin is a good source of health benefits. Gelatin

* Can be a wonderful source of collagen in your diet.

* Contient certain amino acids that can help to build muscles

* Helps maintain joint health

* Helps to balance intake of amino acids
* Promotes growth hormone production
* Helps to increase hair, skin and growth of nails
* Improves digestion
* Improves the health of your gut
* Enhances mood
* Strengthens bones
* Aids in maintaining the cardiovascular health
* Makes you feel full
* Restore firmness to skin that is sagging
* This is a suggestion to help remove cellulite

Gelatin can be used to create amazing culinary applications as well. By adding it to recipes, you can enhance their taste and increase the texture. Did you notice how wonderful the texture of traditional broth compared the canned version? This is because traditional stock has more gelatin.

Collagen is different from. Gelatin - The Differences

Hydrolysed collagen, also known as collagen hydrolysate, is processed more quickly than gelatin. The intense processing of collagen's proteins breaks them into smaller versions of them.

Both gelatin and collagen contain similar amino acids however, they have different chemical ratios.

When it is mixed with water, gelatin is a gel-like substance while collagen doesn't.

In the kitchen gelatin can be more beneficial than collagen.

The main difference between gelatin and collagen comes down to their processing methods. This is the reason for their various appearance, benefits for health and allows them to be treated in various ways.

Similarities Between Collagen And Gelatin

Gelatin and collagen are comparable in that they have the exact amino acid profile since they originate from the same source. A majority of the amino acids present in both of them are anti-inflammatory, making them excellent for general well-being and health.

Both collagen and gelatin have amino acids proline and glutasamine together with glycosaminoglycans which are proteins. They promote the growth of cartilage and improve joint health. This means less joint pain.

Glycine is another link between gelatin and collagen. It is an amino acid that is a potent natural anti-inflammatory component that has the added benefit of supporting the health function of our nervous system as well as enhancing sleep quality and improving the intestinal liner.

Take Collagen as well as Gelatin Supplements

The recommended daily intake of gelatin and collagen powder supplements is 2 teaspoons daily.

Ideally it is recommended that you consume gelatin in the form of a supplement (such as the bone broth in a cup or a teaspoon of collagen in the smoothie in a glass) at every meal you consume throughout the day. Gelatin can be added to soups, sauces, puddings and desserts.

The hydrolysed gelatin powder can be mixed into any liquid. If you purchase gelatin at the grocery store it will likely be available in powders, sheets or Granules.

It is recommended to buy gelatin and collagen products made from grass-fed or pasture-raised animals. They are generally healthy and are not fed antibiotics or synthetic hormones.

Make sure you buy pure, unflavored, organic gelatin every time you are able.

It is important to note that the taste texture and flavour could differ from one kind of gelatin to another and those you can buy in the supermarkets with different flavors aren't always nutritious or full of nutrients.

Gelatin and collagen both offer a number of health benefits which can be maximized by including them in our diets every day and continue to maintain an overall healthy way of life.

After that, we'll continue into the following chapter, where we will discuss the collagen triple Helix.

Collagen Triple Helix

"One of the most important lessons from all of biochemistry
molecular biology and cell biology is the fact that proteins are formed when cells
They operate at the sub cellular level, they behave an arranged manner
as if they're mechanical machines."
James Rothman

The collagen triple-helix, sometimes referred to as the type-2 Helix, is an important shape. It is formed from the repeated sequence of amino acid Glycine - X-Y. The X and Y in this case are proline or proline or hydroxyproline. The hydroxyproline group, generally found in the Y-position is also a stabilizing effect. Due to their repetitive nature collagen chains are prone to be misaligned during folding.

Recent advancements in the study of peptide models have added more clarity to the the structure and function that the triple-helix collagen collagen. If the chain of polypeptides adopts the extended helical structure The three chains get hydrogen-bonded.

The triple-helix motif has been identified in other proteins, other than collagens. It is not only an important structural component and a structural component, it's been recognized as an important component in a variety of biological interactions.

However, the precise extent to which the triple helices interact with one another, could differ from the globular proteins. The triple helix is able to bind domains composed of linear sequences that are arranged along the helix. This makes them receptive to characterisation.

The phosphorylation process of the collagen triple helix can be very crucial for collagen synthesis within the body. It also plays a crucial part within the immune system.

Use

Triple Helix Collagen powder is perfect for healing draining wounds because of its ability to absorb large amounts of fluid. It can take in as much up to 40x its mass of drainage. This is the reason why wound dressings are constructed out of pure collagen.

Triple helix collagen reacted to the extracellular matrix of the skin , and stimulates the production of macrophages and fibroblasts. The body is not able to discern the difference between collagen from within and external, therefore triple helix enhances its capacity to accelerate the healing process.

It is able to be mixed together with wound gel in order to permit access to tunneling wounds. The product is biocompatible (meaning it does not cause negative or toxic effect on live tissue) and is easily absorbed by your body.

Collagen and Whey

"You never have to be old to be younger!"

Mae West

Many search for the perfect wine, while others search are looking for the perfect home and others put in a significant amount of time and effort trying to find the most effective methods to keep young. For those people, nutritious protein and protein supplements are an everyday reality. There's not enough time in a day for them to absorb all the protein that they require to stay young.

While there are a variety of sources of digestible proteins available on the market, they are often contaminated with added ingredients. Additionally, it is the case that they're extremely processed, which takes away the majority of the nutrients, making the protein hard to digest by your body.

Protein from whey has a lot in the same way as collagen. Collagen offers additional advantages in terms of improving your gut health and controlling the metabolism.

But What is Whey?

Whey is one the two major proteins found in milk. It's made from dairy products and it's the fluid released from cheese curds as cheese production begins. In essence, it's the clear liquid appears to be floating on yogurt as you remove the container.

What is the Process Whey Protein Works

A high-quality protein supplement, whey protein will provide you with lots of amino acids that are easily digestible that aid in maintaining the production of collagen within your body. They also aid in slowing the aging process and also serve as the protein that builds muscles.

While it's abundant in amino acids, it's not able to produce the same amount of glycine as collagen. Its high content of glycine helps collagen in treating inflammation better.

Can I Take Collagen and Whey Protein?

Whey and collagen aren't recognized to interact with one another. So, you can take a couple of tablespoons of collagen supplements without worrying about digestive issues or inflammation.

In addition, the additional protein boost from collagen may help you maintain or build muscles when you're working out it doesn't mean you have to lift iron to reap the benefits.

Most people who experiment with collagen love it for its other benefits , including speedier recovery after exercising as well as boosting energy levels and mental dexterity, as well as giving your skin a glowing, healthy glow.

Protein Benefits of Whey Protein Benefits:

* Strengthens muscle mass and assists in weight loss

* Heals the digestive tract.

* Helps reduce appetite

It is easy to take in

Naturally, lower blood pressure naturally

* Can help treat type 2 diabetes

* May reduce inflammation

* Can help lower cholesterol levels.

* Promotes bone health in women

* Enhances the body's antioxidant defenses

* Strengthening the body can be increased.

* Helps reduce stress

* Improves the health of your gut

* Is it anti-cancer?

For those who are lactose intolerant dairy products isn't easy to digest, and it may not provide the same impact on the digestive tract.

Additionally, people who are sensitive to whey may opt for collagen instead.

Different types of Whey

There are five kinds of whey: Concentrate, Denatured and UnDenatured Isolate, Hydrolysed, and Concentrate.

Human breast milk is 60% whey, while cow milk contains 20% Whey.

Protein from Whey is fairly effective and simple to obtain. It can be altered in a variety of ways to produce the desired outcomes. However, a high dose of it could cause diarrhoea, nausea, cramps and so on. It is recommended to use it only as an added supplement to your daily diet.

Collagen Whey Protein

There are collagen-based whey protein supplements available on the market. Make sure you choose one created using grass-fed Whey protein. It must also contain probiotics and natural hyaluronic acids to ensure the best nutrition.

If you exercise regularly or regularly, you may want to consume whey protein and carbs prior to your workout and mix it into smoothies after you have worked out.

Versatility

As with collagen , the whey protein can be added to drinks. You can also add it to plain glasses of water. When it comes to cooking, there are a variety of desserts you can prepare using the whey.

Keep researching and educating yourself on the best ways to include the most protein-rich foods in your diet, without delaying your weight loss efforts. Remember to keep an overall healthy lifestyle to reap the maximum benefits from any supplements.

Cooking using Collagen Recipes

"No illness that is treatable by diet is treatable by diet

must be treated using any other methods."

Maimonides

Healthy living starts by eating a balanced diet. Our bodies thrive when we eat healthy food that is cooked at home. Here are some easy healthy recipes that provide your skin and overall health the boost collagen needs. Some of these recipes can be vegan and vegetarian-friendly too.

Chia Mango Overnight Oats

Ingredients

Chia seeds 1 tablespoon

Chopped mango - 1 cup

Oats in a roll 1/3 cup

Collagen powder 1 heaping tablespoon

1 teaspoon vanilla

Unsweetened almond milk 1 cup

Water 1/2 cup

Cinnamon 1 teaspoon

Cauliflower 1/2 cup

Method

In a smaller saucepan then add the cauliflower. Let it cook for around 4 minutes. Add the oatmeal, collagen powder vanilla, chia seeds cinnamon, and milk. Cook for two minutes, then place it in the bowl, cover it and let it cool overnight.

In the morning, top it with cereal and frozen, or with seeds of your preference. The collagen-rich breakfast is now ready.

Sugar-Free Paleo Collagen Pancakes

Ingredients

Collagen protein powder - 1/4 cup

Medium ripe plantains - 2

Vanilla 1 teaspoon

Shortening the palms of the palms 2 tablespoons

Salt - 1/4 teaspoons

Method

Place all the ingredients in the blender, and mix until it is smooth. Cover a baking dish with parchment. The mixture should be spread 1/4 cup into the baking pan. Bake for approximately 25 minutes at 350 degrees. The delicious sugar-free pancakes waiting for you.

Collagen Chocolate Mousse

Ingredients

Raw cacao powder 2 tablespoons

Full fat coconut milk - 1 can

Collagen peptides - 2 scoops

Cinnamon 2 teaspoons

Method

Cool the coconut milk for a night or up to up to 8 hours. This will break the cream from milk, and bring it to in the middle of the container. Remove the lid from the bottom, scoop the cream out and place it in an mixing bowl. Add the cacao powder as well as cinnamon and collagen peptides to the bowl and mix for approximately 10 minutes. Cool the mixture for about two hours.

Serve chilled and with the freshest fruit or nuts for toppings.

Healing Collagen Tea

Ingredients

Chamomile tea bag 1

Tea bag with peppermint 1

1 teaspoon of turmeric

Collagen powder 1 tablespoon

Boiling water 1 1/2 cups

Vanilla extract - 1/2 teaspoon

Ginger 1 teaspoon

Coconut milk 1 tablespoon

Raw honey 1/2 teaspoon

Black pepper 1 teaspoon

Method

In a large mug of coffee make sure to steep the teas in water for three minutes. Add the remaining ingredients. Mix well, and then take a bite to.

Gummies made of Pomegranate Gelatin

Ingredients

Pomegranate - 1

2 cups of water

Gelatin 4 tablespoons

Stevia or honey - to taste

Method

Bring the water to a boil after which you can add pomegranate and Stevia. Place the lid on and cook for 20 to 25 minutes at medium-high temperatures. Pour the liquid through a strainer in order to get rid of the grains. Place it back on the burner, then add gelatin , and stir it well for a few minutes.

Make sure to grease a few silicone molds using coconut oil. Take the pan off the flame and pour the contents into moulds made of silicone. Refrigerate for about an hour.

Gummies that are healthy and delicious are in the works.

Collagen Deficiency

We share our health and ruin the health of ours."

Jerome K. Jerome K. Jerome

The modern lifestyle has put people at risk of numerous health hazards, such as the risk of obesity as well as type 2 diabetes. It also has resulted in less consumption of collagen that can lead to wrinkles and other indications of aging, as well as joint degeneration.

Around 30% of body proteins are composed of collagen. While the body produces collagen on its own but its capacity to do this decreases as you the advancing years. Thus, the body requires collagen from external sources.

However, due to the diet guidelines that advise us to cut off the skin of chicken and discard the more tough cut of meat we've been collagen-deficient. Deficiency in collagen can cause grave consequences like the loss of skin health, the degeneration of cartilage and joint pain to mention several.

Additionally, it may cause cardiovascular diseases, through the aid of endothelial dysfunction.

It's crucial to recognize collagen deficiency and act accordingly. Here are some signs to look out for.

18.1. Symptoms Of Collagen Deficiency

Since collagen is present in a variety of tissues and organs, it are a variety of signs that suggest the presence of collagen deficiency.

• Wrinkles; loss skin elasticity, skin sagging and skin susceptible to bleeding

The wound heals slowly.

* Frequent muscle pain

* Joint pain, stiffness and joint instability problems.

* Breathing difficulty dry eyes and skin rashes, chest pains and headaches

* Toothache and fallen teeth

18.2. What Can We Do About It?

Vitamin C is an essential ingredient in collagen production. Because our bodies cannot create vitamin C on its on its own, we must supplement the vitamin C needed to gain its advantages. A diet rich in citrus fruits and veggies will assist in sustaining collagen throughout your body.

* Stay away from smoking and excessive exposure to sunlight.

* Choose a diet that is rich in protein from plants.

* Make sure you include plenty of Omega 3 fatty acids in your diet (fish oil, fish and flax seeds)

* Get a good amount of Vitamin D (a minimum of 1000 IU daily)

* Take at least 1000 mg of biotin daily

* Make sure to consume calcium-rich food items (ideal daily intake is 1,000 mg/day prior to menopausal and 1500 mg/day following menopausal transition. It's recommended to take it in a spread in your daily routine, since our bodies aren't designed to take on over 600 milligrams of calcium in one go.)

• Exercise regularly to increase muscle mass to boost the production of collagen.

* Take an assessment of bone density as bones density can be closely tied with collagen (of course, you should consult your physician first)

Collagen injections can also be an option to treat aging and wrinkled skin. The injections are made from animal collagen purified. They are injected into the area affected. Another method to give your body to have a constant amount of collagen can be to take collagen supplements. Consult your doctor should you decide to go for one or the other. Please provide your medical history because the treatment will be specific to your medical history.

Let's look at some beneficial treatments for the skin with simple, DIY collagen masks.

Collagen Face Masks

"I utilize omega-3 oil. I love the feel of light oil for my skin.

It's among my favorite sensations in the world."

Gwyneth Paltrow

Collagen is around 3/4th of the skin, and it assists in keeping the skin's firmness, softness, and softness. To increase collagen levels, you can opt for the costly procedure that requires frequent injections or go for the DIY homemade option by creating your own face masks. Here are five DIY collagen-boosting recipe for face masks.

Moisturising Collagen Mask

Ingredients

5 red grapes

Honey 1 tablespoon

Grapeseed oil or olive oil - 2 teaspoons

How do you create it?

Combine the ingredient until they are smooth. Apply the cream to the face and allow to dry for approximately 15 minutes. Rinse your face with warm water.

Benefits

Red grapes contain resveratrol which is a potent antioxidant that helps to boost collagen production. Olive oil keeps the skin soft and firm.

Prunes and coffee Face Mask

Ingredients

Prunes - 3-4

Coffee powder 1 teaspoon

Water 1 to 3 tablespoons

How do you create it?

In the bowl of a small container, add the ingredients and allow them to rest for around 10 minutes. Mix them up in a food processor and apply the cream to your face. After about 30 minutes, wait and then wash off by using cold water.

Benefits

Prunes are a rich source of antioxidants that help fight wrinkles by encouraging collagen production. Coffee can rejuvenate skin.

Refreshing Collagen Mask

Ingredients

Peach 1. (peeled and purée)

Greek yogurt 3 tablespoons

How do you create it?

Blend the 2 ingredients using the help of a spoon to make the consistency of a batter. Cleanse the face, then apply the cream liberally. Allow it to remain on for around 20 minutes before washing off using warm water.

Benefits

Peaches are loaded with collagen as well as Vitamin C. Greek yoghurt is a superfood of protein. Together, they rehydrate your skin and leave it firm and soft, and provide a pleasant fragrance.

Guava and Carrot Face Mask

Ingredients

Chopped carrot 1/2

Guava chopped and peeled - 1/2

How do you create it?

Combine these ingredients in a blender and blend into a smooth. Apply it all over your face, except for the eyes. Leave it on for 30 minutes. Rinse it off with water.

Benefits

Guava and carrots are both abundant in nutrients like vitamins A, C as well as E. They can help boost collagen production.

Leave-On Collagen Treatment

Ingredients

Freshly squeezed juice of a pineapple 2 tablespoons

Vitamin C tablet - 1 (broken)

1 cup of water

How do you create it?

The ingredients should be heated gently in a pot on a low heat. Allow them to dissolve completely. Refrigerate until the mixture has chilled. Apply it to your face using an unscented cotton ball and allow to dry. Rinse off after a few minutes using warm water.

Benefits

If you don't have vitamin C collagen isn't formed. You must boost the vitamin C levels in your skin for collagen production. Combining tablets with vitamin C and freshly squeezed pineapple juice can be a clever way to achieve this.

Simple, natural DIY collagen treatments will boost the capacity of your skin's cells to produce collagen and benefit from the power of vitamins. The great thing about these treatments is that they can be prepared at home, using ingredients you can readily find in your kitchen.

You've learned almost everything you need that you need to learn about collagen it's time to determine whether there are things as side effects of collagen. We'll now move to the last section.

Collagen Side Effects

"Safety first and foremost is safety."

Charles M. Hayes

As the skin begins to the process of aging, its structure begins to degrade. The body produces lesser and less collagen. However, collagen production can be maintained with the correct supplements. Supplemental collagen can increase the strength of the areas of your skin that wrinkles begin to appear. It can also strengthen the structure of your skin, improve pores and reduce the wrinkles and sagging in the appearance of your skin. This means that you will have healthier, more youthful skin.

How Do Collagen Supplements Work?

Collagen is a naturally occurring protein found in our bodies. It is vital to ensure that skin fibers are tightly together and allows the skin to recover after being pulled. The collagen supplements supply our body with the necessary elements needed to repair tissues.

The supplements are generally derived by consuming animal tissues. After consumption the body breaks them down into peptides as well as amino acids. They are available as creams, pills or lotions, as well as injections. But, prior to taking any supplements, it is important to be aware of the potential negative side effects associated with collagen supplements and treatments.

Incidious Side Effects

Effects on the body can differ based on the type of collagen treatment that you've decided to go through. Collagen creams tend to be expensive and expensive however they don't necessarily have any side negative effects. Collagen supplements taken orally, such as pills, etc. could be dangerous if you suffer from allergies, food sensitivities or other.

There are some side effects from collagen injections including skin allergies. Patients with autoimmune disorders may suffer from flare-ups as the body reacts to foreign substances.

Sometimes an increase in calcium levels in the body may be a result associated with collagen-based supplements. Marine collagen supplements typically cause the issue because they are typically high in calcium. A high level of calcium in the body can cause bone pain nausea, constipation and constipation. They also trigger irregular heart beats. If you frequently take calcium supplements, you must be cautious about supplementing with collagen and seek advice from your doctor.

Hypersensitivity reactions can represent one negative results from collagen supplementation. Based on the National Institute of Allergy and Infectious Diseases hypersensitivity reactions manifest as an abnormal reaction to the immune system allergens, such as foods medications, chemicals and supplements.

Some collagen supplements taken orally may cause unpleasant taste in your mouth. This is treated with fruit juice. Just drink a glass freshly squeezed fruit juice if experiencing this issue and it will go away.

If you're considering taking collagen supplements, specifically oral supplements, bear in your mind that the supplement industry is not among the best tightly controlled industries around the globe. It's difficult to determine the effectiveness of the supplement you've selected for yourself. Talk about the options with your doctor according to your medical history, and continue to maintain your healthy way of life. Start your day early, eat a healthy breakfast and workout regularly. You'll notice the results quickly enough.

Chapter 12: Collagen Breakdown

And Ways To Protect It

"The Most Effective Foundation You Could wear is a radiant healthy skin"

Five Factors Causing Collagen Breakdown

Being one of the primary elements of our skin collagen is what can make our skin virtually impervious to damage when we're young. When we enter the 40s, signs of aging begin to appear and, they bring about all sorts of skin issues like wrinkles, sagging skin as well as decrease in elasticity. When you're exposed to certain triggers it can become a more severe issue (potentially earlier). Let's take a look at the top five causes that cause collagen to break down inside your body.

Stress

Although you may be working in a stressful environment but it's important not to bring your work with you. Stress over time can cause tension in the muscles, which makes it hard to allow your skin and muscles to stay in shape. You should take breaks frequently throughout your day even if for just five minutes, to ease any tension in your tendons and muscles (Kahan and co. 2009).

Age

The body naturally produces less collagen as we get older. The majority of women suffer from a loss of skin elasticity after 50 years. Other factors like smoking and UV rays also play an important role ageing is a fact of life. However, there are actions you can take today to ensure your skin stays well-maintained, even as it gets older daily by using a quality lotion; use sunscreen consistently as well as eat a lot of fruit and drink plenty of fluids and eat foods rich in antioxidants. Choose natural products for your body that do not contain harsh chemicals like parabens or sodium lauryl Sulfate (Varani et al. 2006).

Sun Exposure

The constant exposure to UV radiation can cause irreparable harm to your skin However, you can lessen your risk of developing aged spots and wrinkles keeping your time being in the direct light of. Wearing a high-sPF sunscreen, or better yet, protective clothing that can stop 95 percent or more of harmful UV rays. The darker your skin's complexion is, the greater the amount of sunscreen you require SPF 15 should suffice for the trick for lighter complexions. If you're extremely dark-skinned or have a tendency to burn, you should try applying an SPF of 30 (Bernstein and colleagues. 1996).

Smoking

Smoking cigarettes isn't good for your skin and it's not. Smoking causes wrinkles and prematurely aged skin, however it can also cause hair loss smoking, which makes people who smoke more likely to suffer hair loss due to a variety of causes. The research has found that smoking cigarettes is associated to collagen breakdown across all areas in your body. The chemicals found in cigarettes also weaken teeth and nails by destroying collagen on the surfaces. There aren't quick fixes to repair the damage caused by smoking for a long time. It requires time to allow your body, and your face to improve when you quit smoking entirely.

Poor Diet

Dietary deficiencies affect the overall health of your body and, in particular, its capacity to shield itself from damaging bacteria, harmful toxins, and repair itself. If your diet lacks specific nutrients, then you might suffer from nutritional deficiencies that can cause disruption to many biological processes like collagen production. The collagen could break down if you're not eating sufficient protein, as it could be needed to fulfill different functions.

So, make sure the balance of your food and diverse that includes plenty of fruits as well as vegetables. Also, you should include starchy carbohydrates lean protein, and nutritious fats.

12 Methods to Conserve Collagen

Many people think of beauty or skincare items when hearing collagen. Did you know that collagen affects more than only the skin's surface? It can also help keep various other parts that make up your body look youthful and healthy, including hair follicles, and joints of your legs and arms.

1.) Take in enough Calcium

While you might not consider your body's skeleton as a system for storage it is exactly the case. It can store as much as 30 percent of the total calcium in your body! Once you're over 25 it is recommended to start taking 1,200 milligrams per every day. Why? Because , while your bones expand in adolescence, they don't keep growing forever. Therefore, after the age of 25 years, if you don't absorb sufficient calcium (or vitamin D) via diet or supplements gradually lose bone mass.

2.) Add Minerals

Silica, a common mineral used in cosmetics such as hair conditioners, may help to preserve collagen in your body. Studies have proven that silica can help retain collagen in the skin , helping it remain flexible and firm. If you're seeking various ways to maintain your youthful skin include a healthy supplement made of silica to your diet. But don't expect immediate results. Keep up with a regular routine of incorporating silica and other minerals in your routine if you wish to avoid wrinkles.

3) Lift Heavy Weights

Research suggests that lifting large weights in as little as 12 weeks can boost collagen production. Training with weights for strength doesn't mean you need to lift barbells. Bodyweight exercises like push-ups, planks, squats and pull-ups are equally feasible. There are classes you can begin with if you're just beginning to get started in fitness. If you're interested in learning more about weightlifting, or know how to begin with it, you can contact the local gym or your university's sports department.

4.) Be hydrated

Water is an essential component of an active lifestyle. It's essential for keeping your the skin looking youthful, and it is a source of nutrients for your body. If you're not drinking enough water, you may be dehydrated and result in dry skin and wrinkles. A majority of adults require 13 cups or 2 daily liters of water however, listen to your body's needs. You may require more or reside in a hot climate.

5) Eat Protein

Protein keeps skin solid by forming muscles. A lot of people aren't getting enough protein, and do not have enough collagen production within their bodies. The absence of collagen weakens the skin, which makes it susceptible to wrinkles. The general rule of thumb is 1g protein for every 2 pounds in body mass.

Proteins can be found in lean meats, like chicken breasts or tuna, turkey breast and fish like salmon and cod. Eggs are also a great source of protein, provided that you limit your consumption to 2 eggs each day, as too they can raise cholesterol levels, which could cause health issues later in the future, such as plaque accumulation within your arterial.

6) Sleep well and get Quality Sleep
One of the most important functions is to provide the structure of our body and skin. The body naturally produces human growth hormone, which is a potent anti-aging hormone which maintains the elasticity of our tissues when you sleep. Even if you have a restful night's sleep, you could be putting your skin's health at risk research has shown that not enough sleep can increase cortisol levels, which is your stress hormone that causes an increase in wrinkles on the face (Leproult and co. 1997). For your face to look youthful be sure to have enough rest each night, at least at least eight hours.

7) Eat healthy fats

Certain fats -- like omega-3s from nuts, fish and seeds -- support the skin's ability in maintaining collagen. If you're not getting sufficient healthy fats your body can reduce collagen stores in order to meet demand. Here are some ways to boost the amount of healthy fats you consume:

Consume two portions of fish that are fatty every month (one serving is roughly three pounds)

* Mix ground flaxseed or chia seeds to your morning smoothie

Add chia seeds over the top of your oatmeal or yogurt

* Eat a handful of pumpkin seeds every day high in zinc

8) Take time to be in the natural world

Numerous studies have proven that taking a walk in the fresh air can boost your mood. Not only that, it's completely free! Bring a bit of fresh air to your daily walk by walking outside rather than on the treadmill or stationary bike. Instead from listening to your music consider listening to some bird songs. Listening to the birds' chirping can help reduce anxiety and allows you to be more present.

Any time you devote to the natural world is time to get closer to your own self, so get out and be in nature. It is a great investment both physically as well as mentally.

9.) Let Your Mind Relax

If you're experiencing anxiety at work it may cause a significant strain in your physique. We're all aware of physical signs of stress, such as stomach problems or headaches However, our skin can also be affected. Stress raises cortisol levels which causes dryness, breakouts or uneven complexion leading to weaker collagen. The most beneficial way to take care of our bodies is to know the time to take an interruption from work to unwind our minds and recharge our spirits.

It is possible to avoid the skin problems by making time for yourself. It's more difficult to achieve than it is and if you're unable to take a break from work for a prolonged period or even go outside to take a break, or try meditation or deep breathing prior to when you start your day. It may be a while before you can alter your routine so that you can relax and unwind, but over time it will become routine and most importantly, it will become normal. Even if you do manage to take a break from work completely, pamper yourself time by engaging in activities such as facials or massage therapy to reduce stress levels.

10) Eat Vegetables
If you're trying to preserve collagen, take your meals with lots of vibrant veggies and fruits as you can. Carrots, sweet potatoes lush leaves (like spinach) as well as red peppers, are high of Vitamin C. The greatest benefit? They're also rich in antioxidants, which aid in preventing free radicals from causing harm to your skin. Free radicals are the cause of wrinkles due to the damage that is accumulating over time. Antioxidants counterbalance the effects of free radicals, which means you

won't have to be concerned about wrinkles or sun damage in the future. My top picks are:
* Broccoli
* Kale
* sweet potatoes
* carrots
* oranges
* strawberries
* red peppers
* Apples
* blueberries
* raspberries

Although there are no assurances that these food items will make you look younger Consuming them is a good way to begin preserving collagen right now!

11) Use the Right Type of Product

There are many different items on the market which claim to offer a myriad of things. But, not every product is made to be the same. Instead of seeking out expensive products that claim to increase collagen production, look for ingredients that increase collagen. Prioritizing

ingredients over promises of the marketing, you will be able to benefit from the same anti-aging benefits without the price tag. Be sure to ensure that the products are made up of these ingredients as they have proven to help preserve collagen:
* DNA-repairing enzymes
* Antioxidants
* Peptides

12) Find Professional Help
There are many high-quality skincare treatments available to prevent collagen loss. For instance, you could test:
* Therapy with red light
* Resurfacing with lasers
* Microdermabrasion
* Chemical peels
But, make sure to consult a doctor or dermatologist if you require time to heal or recover from treatments.
4

Avoid Injuries and keep Your Joints Health Y

Do you know how long it takes to recover and fully return to your normal routine If you've been injured. It's good to know that certain supplements can assist in healing quicker than it would otherwise. One of the top ones available that are available today are collagen-based supplements. With collagen, you'll be able to help maintain healthy joints and lower the risk of injuries caused by physical or aging by giving your body nutrients needed to repair itself when it's needed. Continue reading to learn the benefits of collagen, and learn how to assist in recovering quicker from injuries, and stay well-maintained over the long haul!

There are four main reasons for injuries: inadequate training, inadequate preparation for physical exercise and equipment that is not appropriate as well as one's own body (i.e. bones that are weak as well as joints). The cause of injuries can be one incident, such as slipping on the stairs when carrying the laundry basket over time, for instance, in the event that you're not building up your knees because of wear and tear arthritis. It is important to figure the cause to start taking action right away or stop the same thing from happening. If knee injuries seem to keep coming back with no specific trigger for it, consult a physician to have an examination It may be due to low collagen levels.

Collagen is a kind of protein that can help your joints heal faster. The longer you stay away from the joint that is injured or, in certain instances excessively work a healthy joint can affect your joints' capacity to heal. The most common injuries collagen is able to help are joint pain as well as cartilage problems. In these joints, there are cartilage discs which act as shock absorbers to allow your bones to glide across one another when you move. Because collagen is present in cartilage discs it can enhance their function by reducing swelling and pain and speeding up recovery following an injury to the joint.

One of the simplest most cost-effective methods for improving joint wellness is to stock up on foods that are anti-inflammatory. The foods that are rich in dark leafy vegetables are effective in fighting inflammation due to their high content of omega-3 fats (ALA). The vegetables have been proven to decrease inflammation that is caused by chronic illnesses such as lupus, rheumatoid arthritis as well as heart disease, diabetes Alzheimer's disease and Parkinson's disease.

Another great method to improve joint health overall and avoid injury in the future is to take collagen supplements. There are a variety that collagen supplements are available, we'll tell you the information you should know about them:

Hydrolyzed Collagen
Enzymatic processes simply break down the hydrolyzed collagen to smaller, more easily absorbable form known as peptides.

This kind of collagen in liquid form is my favorite and I've seen the greatest results using it (at the absorption level of around 90%)! This supplement is great for nail, skin joints, joints and overall health of muscles.

Collagen Peptides
Collagen peptides are an unflavored, tasteless powder that is able to be mixed with fluids (hot as well as cold) and dissolving without altering the taste. I've used this type of powder previously (different brands) and have not had impressive results, possibly due to the fact that the collagen is a type that has a 77% absorption.

Capsules
Since capsules don't need to be mixed in with liquids or food to consume the only thing you need to remember is to consume them. If you're already taking an supplement program and you're looking for a way to increase your intake, including

a collagen supplement in capsule form is simple to add it.

Gummies

Gummies are like capsules, but they come available in chewable tablet form. It is recommended to stay clear of them as they usually contain excess sugar and calories.

If you're struggling with joint pain, arthritis or tendinitis, including collagen in your diet will help to promote the healing process. The joints of our bodies are comprised of collagen and water which is why it's important to drink enough water. Without adequate hydration joints get stiff and painful, and they aren't as able to heal from injuries. The best way to stay hydrated is to increase your intake of quality protein--particularly protein that contains collagen. It can speed up recovery from injury and ensure your joints are healthy for many years to come.

5

The effects on Collagen Effects of Collagen
Gut Health and weight loss
E
The effects on the effects of Collagen
influence on Gut Health

The health of your digestive system will affect the other parts of your body in many ways, which is the reason it's crucial to keep it in tip-top health. Collagen is often a neglected aspect of gut health but it's got some great health benefits that you need to be aware of to ensure that your gut is healthy and happy.

The digestive tract is usually an area we don't wish to discuss however, it is one of the most important systems. The gut must breakdown food items to ensure adequate nutrition, it helps to keep harmful bacteria out, and ensures that our immunity is top shape. The gut releases hormones, which influence the quality of sleep and mood.

Research has shown that the majority in our body's immune system is within our intestines, so it's not surprising that an endocrine system that is healthy is vital to our general health. If there's a problem with the gut bacteria, we could suffer from constipation, bloating, fatigue, diarrhea, and breakouts on the skin, to mention a few of the signs. In poor health, the gut can be a result due to a poor diet, for example one that is loaded with refined carbs and sugar, as well as lacking important nutrients, like collagen, stress, or lack of sleep. One of the nutrients that play an essential role in maintaining our health is collagen. Collagen is an amino acid that helps support the bones and skin, and assists in digestion as well as various bodily processes.

Numerous studies have been conducted that has linked an imbalanced microbiome to:
* systemic inflammation
* depression, anxiety Other mental health conditions, other mental health and
* recurrent infections, allergies, asthma, autoimmunity

* skin issues (acne, eczemaand psoriasis and more)
* hormonal disorders
* Insulin resistance, cravings and weight increase
* heart problems
* postnatal and prenatal problems

As you can observe your digestive tract plays an important component to overall wellbeing. The gastrointestinal tract functions in conjunction with other areas of your body to assist to digest and absorb nutrients convert amino acids into proteins, create insulin to regulate blood sugar levels and to fight harmful bacteria.

If you're having trouble digesting food, or if you notice that your intestines seem to be in constant discomfort, it could indicate that your body isn't getting the nutrients it needs to function optimally, or that there are toxins within your system.

The collagen that is found in the digestive tract assists in repair and improve the integrity of the gut lining because it is a source of amino acids, including glutamine and glycine. These are crucial in the process. Collagen peptides are able to reduce inflammation and improve joints that are tight in intestinal tract. In a study conducted in 2020, it was found that those who were on the collagen peptide diet had a different microbiota and an increase in short-chain fatty acid production. This is a new exciting field of study that has anti-inflammatory benefits and immunomodulatory effects (Chen and co. 2020).

Additionally, if you suffer from an illness such as leaky gut, you're likely to have issues with absorption of nutrients and digestive issues like food particles escaping from the intestinal lining due to leaky gut. If you can increase the amount of collagen you consume and consuming more collagen, you could be able to reduce some of the consequences of a leaky stomach.

The effects of Collagen on weight loss

Weight loss is a complex process that is influenced by a myriad of elements. The most important factor is your food intake. If you eat less than what your body needs and you lose weight, you'll be losing weight. But it's not all about calories and food weight loss is heavily dependent on the overall health of your body. This is a concern for gut health, metabolism, cortisol levels and stress levels, as well as thyroid functioning. If these parts of your body aren't working properly the body may struggle to lose weight , even though it is in a deficit of calories. There are 5 ways collagen may help:

Collagen Boosts Your Metabolism
If you're like the majority of people you're constantly creating and breaking down protein. The majority of it is used for repair and maintenance, but about 1% is used to provide energy. That means a lean person can theoretically burn around 20 calories over the course of one hour sitting on their back about half the amount you'd burn if you had to work out in 30 minutes.

But increasing your intake of collagen will increase your metabolism and increase the creation of muscle tissue, that means less fat and stronger body at the same at the same time! Try including more collagen-rich foods into your daily diet (such as yogurt, bone broth or meat that is grass-fed) to aid in weight loss!

Collagen Reduces Hunger
You can have a desire-free day by increasing the satiety hormones and decreasing the appetite hormones! Collagen is a rich source of amino acids of high quality, called glycine. These amino acids trigger feelings of satisfaction. The study that uncovered glycine's weight loss effects revealed that those that consumed higher amounts of glycine were less hungry, and had lower levels of ghrelin (the appetite hormone) in their blood (Caldow and co. (2016)).

Collagen Improves Gut Health
Gut health and weight loss are closely linked. If the digestive tract is not working

well it will affect everything from the way your body digests food, to the way it regulates your energy levels. Collagen is among the nutrients that contribute to good gut health However, it's also demonstrated to aid in weight loss. It reduces inflammation in the intestinal tissue which helps in slowing down the rate at which food passes through and helping prevent bloating in patients suffering from IBS, also known as irritable bowel syndrome. (IBS).

In addition, the health of your gut can trigger cravings and hunger in the event that it's overflowing of harmful bacteria. But, because collagen helps bring the equilibrium back (as stated earlier) it regulates hunger and appetite and help your body consume less.

Collagen Helps Build Muscle
If you're trying to start losing weight and maintain it Part of the process is working out and gaining muscles. It's not just about being more attractive - it's about

increasing your metabolism as well as increasing your fitness by strengthening your the tendons and bones, as well as being more confident. To build muscle, your body needs protein. High-quality collagen is a great source of protein that can help to lose weight while building muscles at the same time. A high protein diet with collagen supplements can be a method for dieters to ensure that they don't lose lean muscle mass and lose weight (Zdzieblik and co. in 2015).

Other methods to lose weight
As well as collagen supplements There are a myriad of ways to boost weight loss. For instance, one proven method is to eat regularly throughout the day. Inability to eat regularly results in your blood sugar to vary, which can lead to cravings, and then overeating later in the day. In order to shed weight quickly and safely make sure you eat smaller portions of food every couple of hours. Around every 3 hours is an ideal goal. Combining protein with complex carbs can also reduce your

hunger since it keeps blood sugar levels in check and allows you to feel fuller for longer. Studies have shown that people who consume more protein are likely to weight less than people who consume too much!

Another effective method is exercising. Regular exercise helps you burn off more calories and increase muscles that are lean, accelerating metabolism and helping you eat better. Simple as getting up and taking an easy walk after every meal is just one of the easy ways to incorporate exercising into your daily routine. Other ways to exercise include making frequent breaks from working or during your commute or parking further away from the stores you shop at and setting short-term goals for yourself. For instance, taking a walk to visit a friend's house instead of driving every time!

6

Sun Security Strategies in preparation for Hot Sunny Days

F

I Sun Protection Tips for Hot Sunny Days

When you're running through the woods, laying out at the beach or simply taking a break from summer It's crucial to keep in mind that you're always at risk of sun-related damage or skin cancer, not just on darkest days of the season. There are many ways to reduce the risk even if you're out all day long by protecting your skin with clothes and sunscreen, to having additional protection with sunglasses and caps. These sun protection tips can help you remain safe in the sun even on a hot summer day.

1.) Put on a Shade Hat

A wide-brimmed hat could be an absolute lifesaver during the hot days of summer. It helps to keep cool while shielding your face from the direct sun and also prevents overheating. The greater the area of your body that remains cool more, the longer you'll remain outside in the scorching heat.

2.) Don't spend any time in direct UV light

UVA and UVB sun's rays could cause damage to the skin such as wrinkles, sunspots, and uneven coloration. Be sure to protect your face by wearing sun hats that have brims that cover your neck and face in the event that you have to be outdoors. Also, sunscreen that has SPF at least 30 is recommended to be applied to all exposed skin areas within 15 minutes prior to leaving.

3.) Increased Intake of Collagen Peptides
The sun's ultraviolet radiation breaks down collagen, one of the body's most abundant natural sources of skin-plumping proteins. To ensure that your skin is able to take this pounding, consider taking an antioxidant supplement with collagen. Collagen helps to create new cells, which helps keep wrinkles at bay as well as keeps elasticity intact, making it an integral part of any anti-aging skin care routine. Find gel caps that contain the molecule hyaluronic acid. Its molecules are small enough to penetrate deep into the skin to boost the

amount of moisture (which helps to increase the production of collagen).

4.) Wear protective clothing
Clothing that shields your skin can stop UV radiation from reaching the skin and reflecting away. Although loose-fitting clothes are more likely to result in the exhaustion of heat, tight dark shades provide no protection against ultraviolet radiation. Opt for lighter shades such as yellow and white that reflect the majority of UV radiation that is harmful to the sun. Another alternative is wearing long-sleeved shirts and pants. Just remember to apply sunscreen every time you put them on. Although wool-like fabrics protect against UVA Rays, they don't provide protection against UVB radiation. Additionally, they are more likely to cause itching during warm weather.

5.) Use Sunscreens
Beware of sunscreens that leave behind an opaque white film or pores-clogging properties If you are a fan of tanning.

Choose a broad-spectrum sunblock that has an SPF of at minimum 30. Find ingredients such as avobenzone (also called Parsol 1789) and Mexoryl SX that offer excellent protection from UVA Rays. Chemical sunscreens made of synthetic chemicals protect your skin from UV radiations that are the primary causes of premature aging Melanoma and various forms of skin cancers. Consider avoiding organic chemical sunscreens, as they could not offer enough protection against UVA radiation. Avobenzone is the best choice.

7

Boost Your Collagen Levels

10 Tips to Increase Your Collagen Levels

As of now, you've discovered a lot about collagen and its functions. In this section we'll take a look at ten strategies you can make use of to boost the production of collagen. This is extremely beneficial in the event that you're already at a point in a situation where collagen stores be diminished.

1.) Get more Vitamin C.

Vitamin C plays an essential part in the production of collagen which is why your skin can be affected if you don't get enough of it from your diet. The green tea and oranges are among the most abundant food sources for Vitamin C. This superfood is able to improve your skin's condition and keep it looking fresh as you get older (Pullar et al. 2017, 2017). If you aren't a fan of oranges, or any other fruit that is citrus, excellent sources are the kiwis, strawberries, and cantaloupe. The recommended daily intake of vitamin C is 75 mg for women and 90mg for males however certain studies have demonstrated that higher doses can aid in fighting diseases by encouraging growth of white blood cells.

2.) Apply Retinoid to Your skin

Retinoids are vital to collagen production since they stimulate the fibroblasts. The best source of retinoid is prescription-strength tretinoin (found in Retin-A,

Renova, and Avita). However, you can get it in non-prescription anti-aging creams that contain vitamin A derivatives, such as retinyl Palmitate (found in a variety of products by SkinCeuticals, Alpha Hydrox, and Neutrogena). The ingredients in these products boost collagen production and help keep the rate of turnover in your skin high and results in a more smooth appearance, thanks to the fact that pores are kept clear.

3) Massage Your Skin

Massage is a quick and easy way to boost collagen production within your routine. Massage improves blood circulation. This is beneficial for general skin health however, it also improves lymphatic drainage which can rid your body of the toxins and waste materials. This can help keep your skin looking and feeling healthy.

4.) Bone Broth

In order to ensure your protein intake is sufficient into your diet, and to load with nutrients that strengthen your bones, try drinking the equivalent of a cup of broth each day. In addition to being packed with protein, it also contains collagen-boosting minerals and nutrients. For instance beef bone broth has the healthy amount of Vitamin K2 which is crucial for our bones since it assists in transferring calcium into the bloodstream. Bone broth can be made using chicken or fish bone instead of beef which makes it a viable alternative for vegetarians too.

5) Cleanse regularly

Make use of a body scrub like one that is made of sugar or salt , to scrub out dead skin cell. The dead skin cells represent your body's way of telling you to let me go. It is possible to keep them in check by not exfoliating frequently and not over-moisturizing. Exfoliation also helps keep the same color and helps keep all other anti-aging treatments in place. Make sure to exfoliate at least once per week for the most effective results.

Cleanse your skin using an circular motion. Make a body scrub by combining sugar or salt, mixed with body temperature water. gently massage it on your skin. Exfoliating isn't just an easy method to boost collagen production naturally , but is also quicker than other anti-aging treatments.

6) Micro-needling

Micro-needling is a well-known method for those who are unhappy with their aged skin to have younger skin. It involves rolling a small handheld device that appears like the shape of a pen on your face. While you roll the needles, they create tiny holes in the skin which prompt your body to boost collagen production. This treatment can help reduce the appearance of redness, as well as other signs of aging, as well as wrinkles and fine lines. It could even help reduce the appearance of scars.

7) Collagen Supplements

As we get older, collagen levels decrease, and supplementing with a supplement is an affordable and cost-effective option to increase the collagen levels in our bodies. Keep in mind that various collagen supplements are made differently and can have different effects. The most commonly used types in supplements are those that are hydrolyzed (processed using water) and gelatinized (processed with very high temperature). Amino acids, the protein building blocks can also be added to create an all-inclusive collagen supplement. If you choose to take supplements over foods that are that contain collagen sources, search for one that contains vitamin C. It can increase the absorption.

8.) Eat plenty of Omega-3s

Human bodies aren't able to produce omega-3 acid fatty acids. But it is able to convert some essential fats into them. Two of these fats are alpha linolenic acid (ALA) and the stearidonic acid (SDA). But, this process is not efficient, and we need to consume omega-3s all throughout our meals. The best sources of omega-3s are the fat-rich fish like mackerel and salmon. If you are a plant-based eater or wish to avoid taking in large quantities of fish ought to consider supplementing by eating plant-based omega-3s rather than hemp seeds, for instance.

9) Chia Seeds
One of the most effective source of collagen is chia seeds. They aid in increasing your intake of skin-enhancing, hair-nourishing nutrients. When you switch out your the traditional breakfast cereals and oatmeal in favor of a more nutritious breakfast bowl with chia seeds as well as oatmeal--which is a great supply of starch that is resistant which is beneficial for gut health, you'll give your body an easy method to boost the amount of collagen you consume.

It aids in firming loose skin, and also prevents stretch marks from your stomach, breasts the thighs, and your rear! Chia seeds also are extremely hydrating. They're over 90 percent of water in weight. The moisture in the air can to soothe dry hair and skin and strengthen your bones.

10) Sculptra Injection

A needle is not an option for me because I am not a big fan of needles. But, you can improve the collagen levels of your body through non-surgical injection treatment. Sculptra is also known as poly-L lactic acid is an injectable that is similar to Botox (by briefly paralyzing certain muscles) However, it has some significant advantages. The injections can increase collagen production, leading to an increase in volume in your face and a more youthful look. Due to the fact that Sculptra is more durable in comparison to Botox (about 2 years, compared up to 3 months) It's also less costly in the long run.

Chapter 13: Collagen Protein: What Is It?

The name Collagen originates from a combination of its Greek word kolla meaning "glue" as well as"glue," and French word -gene which means "something that creates". Collagen is an amino acid that gives the body structure and keeps the body in place.

Every sq inch in our body is a source of it, making it the largest protein. It essentially functions the same way as it is a "glue" that keeps the body in place. (Animals also utilize collagen to accomplish the same purpose and that's what makes them the primary source of collagen found in your diet.)

To be more precise (by dry weight) collagen is comprised of:

1. 10% to 11% of the muscle mass
* 90 90% of the sclera (the white portion in your eye)

* 70%-80 percent of the skin
* 80percent of tendons
* 60 60% of cartilage
* 30 percent of bones

In general there are the various kinds of collagen present within connective tissues.

A Comparative Study of the various Kinds of Collagen
The body's collagen is composed of at least 16 different types however, between 80 and 90% is composed from collagen type I, II and III.

* Collagen I The most abundant collagen protein is of type 1. Tendons, skin, bone connective tissue, cartilage and even teeth all are made of collagen. Because collagen fibrils of type I are extremely durable they are able to withstand massive quantities of pressure. No matter what stress they're put under they won't break. The collagen is so strong that it is able to outperform steel, gram forgram.

* Collagen II -- Most cartilage has this type of collagen. The type 2 collagen form is vital for joint healthand that is the reason it helps prevent the onset of structurally-based arthritis-related joint pain.

* Collagen III It is also another important kind III that is found in muscles organs, arteries and organs and also a specific type of connective tissue known as reticular fibre (which is a structural component that supports the liver, adipose tissue bone marrow and spleen). Research on animals suggests that collagen deficiencies can increase the risk of ruptured blood vessels as well as early death.

* Other than collagen type I and III, the other types of collagen that can be present within the body (although less frequently than types I-III) are type IV, V and X.

* Collagen IV -- Underneath the epithelium this type creates the basal lamina which is a layer of extracellular matrix (the tissue matrix that provide support to cells). Skin cells are supported externally through the lamina basal.

* Collagen V -- A form of collagen known as collagen V can be found in the corneas, bone matrix, and connective tissues surrounding the liver, muscles the lungs, and the placenta (also called"the interstitial matrix).

* Collagen X -- forming new bones and articular cartilage are assisted by the type X. The endochondral osteossification occurs in the course of. In addition to healing of the healing of synovial joints, it is well-known that it helps in the process of the regeneration of tissues.

The main difference between different types of collagen can be found in the proteins (amino acid chains) which create the chains. Collagen is different in its forms and properties based on the peptides it contains and the way they connect.

What is the composition of Collagen?
Amino acid, the basic protein blocks, form the peptides (which we've discussed in the

past). A proper mix of amino acids essential for a protein's function to fulfill its purpose. The body produces different kinds of proteins, each serving different functions.

As compared to any other proteins, collagen has the highest amount of proline and Glycine, than any of the other amino acids. Both amino acids are regarded as "conditionally necessary," which means that the body produces these two amino acids, but only in small amounts and in certain conditions.

The body produces them in normal times, but it stops producing them when it is sick or under stress. So, collagen powder and the bone broth is considered to be dietary sources of collagen when they are taken to reap the maximum health benefits.

The answer to this question "What are the main components that make up collagen?" To discuss collagen's structure more detail, here's an easy description of its general to specific components:

* Collagen -A fibrous substance composed of collagen.
* Amino acid -- The body's proteins are constructed from these components. Glycine and proline are the primary elements of collagen.
* Peptides Every protein is made up by amino acids chains. These amino acids make up the collagen chains.

Since collagen is made up of components (amino acids) we will look at the way collagen is constructed.

Collagen and the Making of Collagen

There are three primary steps in the production of collagen:

1: Procollagen

Collagen is an elixir of procollagen. The protein is made up of three amino acids. It is designed to look like three helixes:

* Proline
* Glycine (about 30 percent of collagen's amino acid)
* Hydroxyproline

The majority of procollagen helixes contain this sequence: Gly-X-Y (Proline as well as Hydroxyproline is generally two X as well as Y).

There are a variety of additional amino acids not related to collagen chains, which comprise:

* Glutamic acid
* Arginine
* Lysine
* Alanine

Based on the location where amino acids are located in the chain and the type of amino acids that are within the chain.

Collagen will be made and what particular characteristics it has.

A variety of chemical changes are caused by the endoplasmic retina (ER) that produces a procollagen chain that is brittle. Phase 1 concludes with the final product.

Within the Golgi apparatus (a vesicle in the collagen-forming cells) the procollagen chain gets added to the oligosaccharides (complex carbs). Then, it's packaged and then released outside the cell.

2. Tropocollagen

Once procollagen has been removed from the cell, it gets separated from the cell in an area known as the extracellular space. Collagen strands or tropocollagen, are the result of this process.

3: Collagen Fibril Formation

A collagen protein is composed by fibres made from tropocollagen (collagen strands).

If you were to describe the collagen manufacturing process you could picture the process as plying rope comprised from three threads. It is made up of chemicals that allow the strands to connect, by helix-twisting them into a single strand, leaving the ends sagging, which are then cut and closed. The collagen forms at the conclusion of this process.

What is it that makes Collagen Different from Other Proteins?
It might be confusing to you after having absorbed all this information about collagen. what it's all about and what it shares with other proteins like meat, fish or whey. The fact that they're all protein sources doesn't alter that fact, does it?

Although all proteins contain amino acids they don't trigger the same physiological reactions. This is due to the fact that before amino acid molecules are able to be used, proteins must be broken down into the component amino acids. In other words the arrangement of amino acids contained in your protein can determine a good amount about how your body utilizes it.

Leucine, an amino acid for instance is a potent stimulator of insulin release and triggers the IGF-1 and the mTOR pathways to function. In the wake of leucine anabolism (tissue growth) is observed.

A large portion of proteins in dairy and meat products is leucine. This is why these proteins are widely promoted as muscle-building substances. But, they could cause cancer cell growth and even outbreaks.

Alongside methionine, an additional amino acid which could cause problems in large amounts is Lysine. Proteins from fish and meat are rich in homocysteine it is an amino acid which could alter the levels in blood of the chemical. Stroke, heart disease and mental illnesses are all a result of excessive homocysteine levels.

The impact of consuming excessive amounts of methionine and leucine over a body that is not active might be the reason why certain studies have found a link between consumption of red meat to heart disease and cancer. In any event changing to a vegan ketogenic diet isn't an solution.

In the event that we consume additional amino acids alongside meat, it is possible to eat meat as part of a balanced diet, without suffering from the adverse health effects of excessive methionine and leucine inside the body. It is understood that glycine and proline - - the two most commonly used amino acids in collagen - combat the negative effects of an active mTOR pathway (due to in part the leucine levels being elevated) and the excessive consumption of methionine.

Fish, meat and dairy products can't compete with the distinct benefits collagen protein can provide advantages that are not present with other protein sources.

Dietary Collagen Benefits from the Keto Diet
Collagen levels are sufficient and eating collagen can provide health advantages. Here are a few outcomes you can observe and feel:

Improves Skin Health and reverses the signs of skin Aging

Rubging collagen onto your skin will not make any difference. In the body, collagen produces profound and lasting effects on the skin. The research has shown that supplementation with collagen (such such as bone or collagen):

* Skin is more elastic

* Collagen is kept from breaking down

* Collagen production is increasing

* Decreases the risk of early signs of the aging process

* Enhances skin elasticity, hydration and flexibility the skin

* Helps to reduce the appearance of aging skin by decreasing roughness

* Causes the skin to produce more collagen.

* Guards against UV-induced damage Reduces cellulite effectively

For these benefits to be felt What amount of collagen is needed? At present, there's only sufficient evidence to suggest the dosage of 1/2 to one tablespoon collagen hydrolysate (or any among the collagen supplementation options we'll to explore in the near future) is adequate. To get the other benefits that collagen offers, it might require a higher daily dose.

Maintains a Solid Nail

The negative effects of the intake of collagen through oral intake on our nails were discovered in a study:

* The rate of growth of nails was increased by 12 percent.
A decrease of 42% of broken nail fractures was recorded.
After 4 weeks, the integrity of the nail was significantly improved.

Reduces Hair Loss Due to Premature Growth

Apart from maintaining your nails' strength and healthy, collagen can also help reverse the signs of loss of hair. The study conducted in Journal of Investigative Dermatology revealed an the extracellular matrix (ECM) is a major part in shaping hair follicle growth and may suggest that collagen VI might be a viable remedy for loss of hair as well as other skin issues.

Although research on this subject is not a lot, it's possible that giving your body the nutrients and vitamins required to create collagen can prevent hair loss.

Increases Muscle Growth and Recovery
The same way as other proteins are essential in the growth of muscles and for recovery, collagen is important for healing and growth. When collagen is supplemented it is able to:

* Strengthening muscles
* Enhance the efficiency of resistance training
* Rejuvenate muscles
The condition of the muscle are preventable

In a research study, which examined collagen supplementation in conjunction with resistance training for sarcopenic older males, supplementing collagen improved the muscle mass and strength as well as reducing the amount of fat that

173

accumulates. Collagen improves the strength of muscles and strength for men who have difficulty maintaining their muscle mass.

However, collagen VI deficiency can affect muscle regeneration and lower the capacity for cells to self-renew following injuries.

The optimal health of Joints, Tendons, and Ligaments

Tendons and ligaments are composed by 80percent collagen. the collagen forms I, II III IV, and XI are most fundamental elements. Therefore, collagen deficiency can result in joint problems, and low flexibility.

Particularly collagen supplementation with peptides has been shown to be:

* Make sure that the ligaments and tendons are in good shape.

* Treat rheumatoid arthritis as well as osteoarthritis with a natural approach. Reduce joint swelling and discomfort.
* Offer support for repair of tendon

Another investigation, random double-blind study involving 60 patients suffering from rheumatoid arthritis discovered that the type II collagen in chickens reduced the amount of joints that were tender and swollen and four patients had complete remission within 3 months.

The results of a second double-blind research study have revealed that collagen peptides can be useful nutritional supplements to treat osteoarthritis as well as maintain joint health.

Enhances Bone Strength
To maintain optimal bone health, you require greater than just calcium.

The combination with calcium calcitonin (a calcium-derived chemical) along with collagen is proven to decrease the breakdown of collagen in the bone better than just calcitonin on its own. The amount of collagen a child consumes affects how their bones develop and are developed at crucial growth stages.

Simply put collagen is a good thing for bone health when it is combined with calcium.

Improves the Health and Overall Well-being of the Tissue
Our wounds wouldn't be healed without collagen. One article in a journal describes the scar as "a powerful collagen filler that helps restore strength and integrity to tissue damaged by tissue damage."

A deficiency in collagen (or an insufficient amount of the essential substances that help collagen production that we'll discuss in the future) can hinder the healing process.

Keeps your eyes healthy Eyes

The Type VII collagen an significant part of the eye, because it is the cornea, the retina and the sclera (the white portion that makes up the eyes). A lack of collagen XVIII can cause eye defects and malformations.

If you're lacking in collagen XVIII you don't have to search for supplements. The body is capable of producing collagen by itself if it gets the amino acids and micronutrients that comprise it.

Gut Health is improved
The gut is repaired and protected by collagen. This is made possible through collagen peptides, which help in the improvement of the integrity of intestinal barrier cells.

It is essential to take this step to keep our health in good shape since the intestinal barrier functions as an obstruction between our blood circulation and the food we consume. Through absorption of nutrients, electrolytes, as well as water your body is protected against pathogens.

Because of a weakening of the wall, intestinal problems like inflammatory bowel disease as well as bleeding gut, celiac disease and diarrhea could develop. There is also the possibility of chronic inflammation when our gut is lacking collagen.

It is due to collagen's potential effects on digestion bones that it is frequently described as an "gut healer." The collagen in bone broth is a rich source of amino acids, which are vital to maintain an encapsulated intestinal barrier that is healthy.

How can you benefit from Collagen
Three strategies need to be employed for maximizing the advantages of collagen:

Make sure you are avoiding the factors in your life that make collagen deplete.

* Be sure to eat foods that are rich in vitamins and minerals collagen requires to make, regulate, and defend its own.

Consume collagen supplements (or supplements containing amino acids from collagen).

The reason you shouldn't benefit of Collagen and what you can do to do

The structure as well as the strength and endurance of your collagen is mostly determined by genetics and aging, however you can alter the following factors:

* Diet high in sugar. It's been found that fructose and glucose can stop collagen from being utilized for repairing our bodies and also cause AGEs within our bodies. Sugar reacts with lipids and proteins to cause AGE, and this toxin can be associated with chronic diseases such as diabetes. If you follow a low-carb, moderate sugar diet, such as that of keto,

you will prevent sugar from affecting the production of collagen and skin.

* Because of the slow production of both type I as well as III collagens, smoking leads to premature facial wrinkles and weak wound healing. It is important to stop smoking completely to stop this from happening and to maintain the optimal collagen production.

* Excessive sun exposure. The health of our entire body needs exposure to the sun, however, excessive exposure to the sun can harm the collagen in our body and slow down collagen synthesis, which makes our skin more fragile. To reap the benefits of the sun will require at least 3 to 30 minutes of midday exposure to the sun that has at least 40% of your skin exposed (people with darker skin types may require more than 30 minutes of exposure to the sun and those with lighter skin might only require only a couple of minutes).
*

Air pollution. There is a thing called particles (PM) in air that is polluted comprised of very small particles that are taken up by your lungs and the skin. After absorption into your skin, particles could cause an oxidative stress, break collagen and increase the risk to develop skin cancer. The best method to avoid these problems is to lower the amount of pollutant that you breathe by (1) shifting to a place with less pollution and (2) making use of air purifiers equipped with HEPA filters.

* Nutritional deficiency. A lack of nutrients that make collagen can cause deficiencies. Nutrition plays a significant role in the prevention of collagen breakdown and in maximising the advantages.

The Best Supplement to Collagen
The following characteristics must be taken into account when searching to find a supplement made of collagen

Derived via the Right Animal
Bovine collagen powder is among the most effective available today. The majority of research has been conducted on bovine collagen, and it's also the easiest to locate.

You can expect better results from this source due to numerous reasons.

Pig collagen is not well-studied and is typically derived from animals that are unhealthy.
* It is recommended to stay clear of chicken collagen since it could be infected with Avian illnesses.
* With their distinct particle size, the marine and fish collagen appear promising, but they're not yet tested and need more study before they are accepted as safe and effective.
* Healthy cows that are fed grass can easily be used to obtain bovine collagen.

Organically-Raised 100% grass-fed
Your health and the planet will be healthier if you consume collagen that is sourced from grass.

A study revealed that animals that eat grass have higher levels of beta-carotene (the precursor to vitamin A, which is derived from plants) in comparison to animals fed grains. Vitamin A is essential to maintain the integrity of the cow's hide which is the principal tissue from which collagen peptides can be created, should be taken into consideration.

This implies that cattle fed with grass have better hides, which could make grass-fed collagen more valuable for us.

If grass-fed and grain-fed collagen is not clearly distinguished using grass-fed collagen gives you sustainable farming methods that is more suited to the natural environment.

Each serving must contain at least 10 grams of Collagen
Hydrolyzed collagen with a dosage of 10 grams per day can benefit joints, skin, and bones (and additionally to that, you could reap certain benefits from Glycine with this dose). To ensure that you get the most benefits out of the supplement you are taking, be sure that you include at

minimum 10% (10,000mg) of grass-fed, pure collagen peptides for each serving.

No fillers are necessary.
Because collagen peptides require only an ingredient that is listed on the product label. the supplement should read something like this:

* Collagen powder that has been hydrolyzed from cattle fed grass
* Collagen peptides that are made from cattle that are fed grass
• Collagen is hydrolyzed by beef

Be sure to stay clear of supplements that contain gelatin, magnesium Stearate, or sweeteners other than stevia or erythritol. A collagen supplement in its pure form will contain only one ingredient and not include carbohydrates or fat.

www.ingramcontent.com/pod-product-compliance
Lightning Source LLC
Chambersburg PA
CBHW060327030426
42336CB00011B/1236

* 9 7 8 1 7 7 4 8 5 7 7 8 6 *